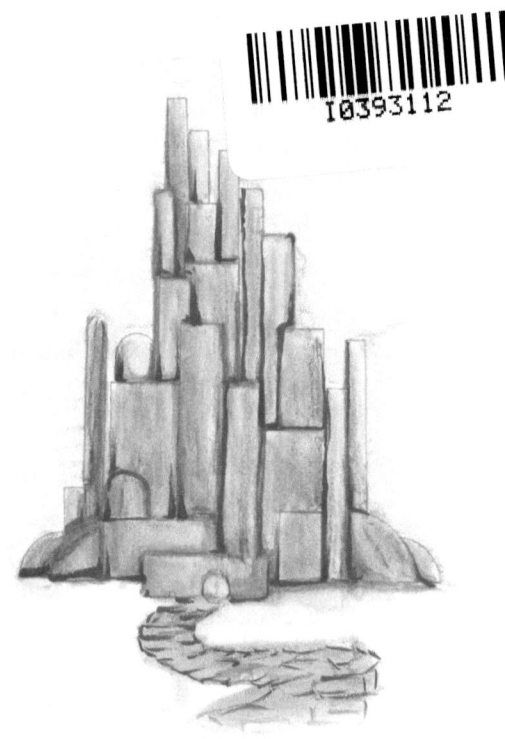

The Yellow "Sick" Road

A Nurse's Travels for 22 Years

A Story of Bullying in the Workplace

Claudia Sanborn
Illustrations by: Bruce Sanborn

The Yellow "Sick" Road: A Nurse's Travels for 22 Years

Text Copyright © 2015 Claudia Sanborn

Illustration Copyright © 2015 Bruce Sanborn

Formatting by: Mikey Brooks (insidemikeysworld.com)

While this book is a work of nonfiction, names of real persons and places have been changed to protect the innocent. The views expressed in this book are those of the author and do not represent the official position of the Utah Heathy Workplace Advocates. Characters used in this book are based off the those depicted in L. Frank Baum's *The Wonderful Wizard of Oz*, part of the Public Domain as of 1923.

No part of this book may be reproduced or transmitted in any form or by any means, electronic or mechanical, including photocopying, recording, or by any information storage and retrieval system without express written permission from the author.

All rights reserved.

Paperback Edition

ISBN-13: 978-1514308882

ISBN-10: 1514308886

Contents

Prelude 1

Chapter One: Cyclone 8

Chapter Two: Flash Cards 17

Chapter Three: Knobby Finger 23

Chapter Four: The Witch's Spell 31

Chapter Five: Emerald City—Illusion 37

Chapter Six: Emerald City—Real 43

Chapter Seven: Dead Daughter 49

Chapter Eight: Emerald City—Falling........... 53

Chapter Nine: The Ditch 65

Chapter Ten: Washington DC 69

Chapter Eleven: The Gypsy 77

Chapter Twelve: The Desk 84

Chapter Thirteen: Pending Doom 94

Chapter Fourteen: Religious Emerald City 100

Chapter Fifteen: The Munchkins 105

Chapter Sixteen: Vase with a Red Carnation 112

Chapter Seventeen: The Confession 117

Chapter Eighteen: Dying 121

Chapter Nineteen: Really Scary 127

Chapter Twenty: Pushing a Bug with a Stick............... 132

Chapter Twenty-One: Legislature................................ 139

There's an Old Sick Road.. 147

Acknowledgments

About the Author

Bibliography

The Characters

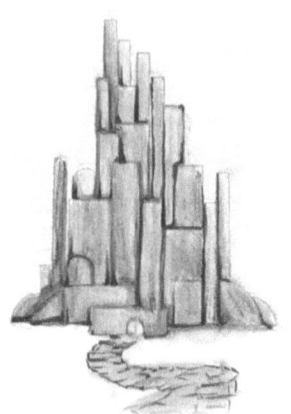

The Emerald City:
The Hospital

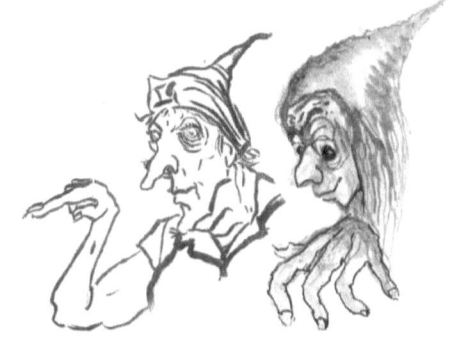

The Witches:
Charge Nurses
& Management

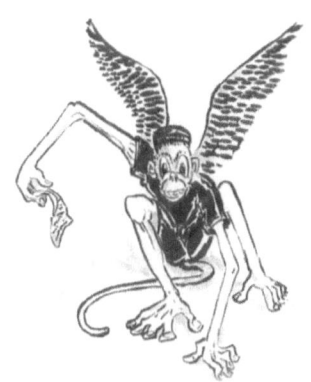

Flying Monkeys:
The Nurse's Aides

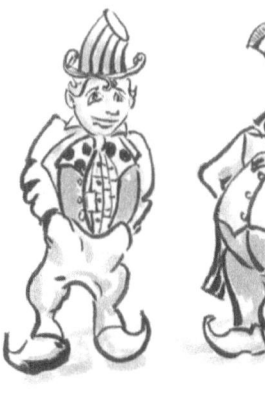

Munchkins:
The Patients

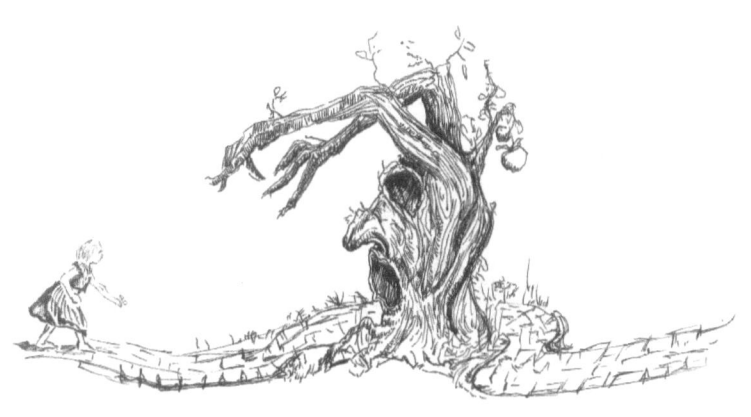

Prelude

Yellow Sick Road

I walked into the elderly patient's room, shocked to see her lying on the floor, naked, covered with blood oozing from a transfusion bag still attached to her arm. I could only guess that her state of dementia had caused her to undress and try to get up by herself while still attached to medical equipment with IV lines.

Where was the aide?

I dropped to my knees and checked to make sure

Prelude

the patient on the floor was stable. I dragged a blanket from the bed and covered her, knowing I couldn't get her back into bed on my own. I called out for the aide, but no one answered.

With no other choice, I left the patient and quickly searched the unit for the aide who was supposed to help me. I was the RN (registered nurse) on duty, and the aide was the only other employee on the premises. As I searched, I grew increasingly panicked, wondering if the patient on the floor had hit her head or broken a bone.

At last I found the aide sitting in a room with the light off, talking on the phone. Not only was I upset that she had not informed me she was taking a break, but I wasn't happy that she seemed to be hiding from me. When I told her I needed her right now, she helped me get the patient back in bed where I did a more thorough assessment, including taking her vital signs. To my relief, the patient checked out okay.

Since the aide's negligence constituted a serious breach of hospital protocol, I reported the incident to the charge nurse/manager the next morning. I expected that my supervisor would agree with me that I should write an Incident Report. To my surprise, she recommended that I not do so. She said I should just let the incident pass.

I was shocked as my supervisor explained that since the aide was an ethnic minority and this was a University Hospital, the aide could claim discrimination. It would likely go clear to the top and turn on me, since I was a fairly new nurse and this was my first job. "You won't stand a chance," the charge nurse told me.

It really bothered me that this aide would suffer no consequences for her thoughtless actions. She wasn't even called in to talk to management about the incident.

After that night, whenever I worked with that aide, it usually felt as if I were taking care of as many as 10-12 patients alone. I would have to toilet and turn patients all by myself, a job that is hard even when you have a good coworker helping. I felt hopeless because it seemed like she could do anything she wanted without having to account to me, her supervisor, for any of her actions. Nursing is supposed to be a team effort, but because of management's aversion to potential racial issues, I was basically a team of one.

Prelude

I want to make it clear that I am not prejudiced against any person or race. I grew up with people of all nationalities and learned to work with everyone. The problem here is that, because of a racial bias not my own, I didn't have support from management over an issue that clearly affected patient care and well-being.

Had the charge nurse and management been taught their correct leadership roles, then the consequences for the aide would have been appropriate and fairly administered.

This is a clear-cut example of why it should be mandatory for management to be educated and certified in how to handle such incidents. They should also be evaluated to assure they have the proper temperament and personality traits necessary to manage hospital staff.

This incident and the others in this book are true. Because I had so many questionable things happen during my twenty-two year nursing career, one of my goals when I finished nursing was to let the public know what really happens in the nursing medical field. Hopefully, you will learn a lot from these pages, and the experiences will give you more understanding of issues related to bullying in the workforce.

In Alexandra Robbins' book, "The Nurses: A Year of Secrets, Drama, and Miracles with the Heroes of the Hospital,"[1] the author used hundreds of interviews with nurses to gather the following statistics:

- 85% of nurses have been verbally abused by a fellow nurse
- 1 in 3 nurses quit because of bullying
- It's bullying, not the wage, that is the major cause of the global nursing shortage (the Bureau of Labor Statistics projects that by 2022, there will be a shortfall of 1.05 million nurses.)
- Many hospital units don't give nurses time to eat, take a walk, or even go to the bathroom.

There are many possible causes for bullying, such as making a new nurse prove herself, overwork, lack of appropriate outlets for built-up frustrations, or inflated egos, but whatever the cause, if health care professionals can't effectively communicate with or support one another, it's the patient who ultimately suffers.

Prelude

For those who want to improve the conditions of the workforce, you must first be aware of what is going on. Become involved with the legislature in your state and vote for bills to be passed that could prevent harm not only to people in the medical field, but in all areas of work.

I've chosen to use the "Wizard of Oz" characters and metaphors to make this story more descriptive, because some things that happened were so surreal. I also feel that a lot of the characters from the book fit well with the different staff members and patients I worked with throughout the years.

"The Yellow Sick Road" explains my journey down a road that was sometimes crooked, sometimes bumpy, and sometimes pleasant. The Witches - East, West, North, and South - represent the charge nurses and management. The nurse's aides are the Flying Monkeys. The Wizard of Oz is the CEO. The lion, scarecrow, and tin man have character qualities and desires that match my own. Emerald City is the hospital, and Dorothy's home is like my home, sweet home whenever I returned from working as a travel nurse for past six years.

There's no place like home.

The Yellow "Sick" Road

I have not held back or exaggerated any of the facts and stories written here. I have also added some incidents from my personal life in order for you to understand my deep desire to be a nurse and where that path led me. I am proud to be a nurse.

"And ye shall know the truth, and the truth shall make you free." John 8:31-32

—Claudia Sanborn RN

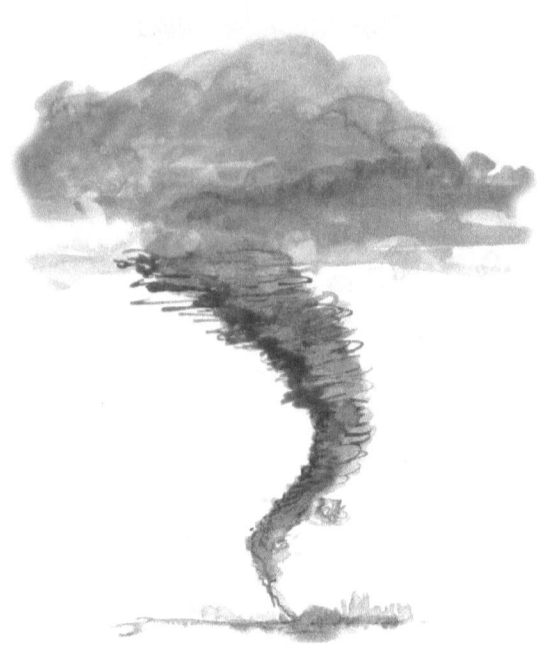

Cyclone

My Life Prior to Becoming a Nurse

Before all of us stretches a Yellow Brick Road of sorts. Everyone born into this world gains life experience along the way. Some spots along the road are pleasant, while others may be bumpy and treacherous. For me, the road has been filled with many unexpected twists and turns.

My life was swept up in a cyclone in 1982 when my husband moved with me and our four sons Jeff,

The Yellow "Sick" Road

Ryan, Scott, Mark to California to pursue a job opportunity. Two years after the move, with 14 years of marriage behind us, he decided to run off with his secretary.

I remember where I was standing when he told me he didn't love me anymore, and that he wanted a divorce. We weren't even fighting. He said it in the most nonchalant, casual way imaginable, and it caught me totally off guard. I looked at him in shock and said, "I don't believe you."

I was a stay-at-home mom who wasn't focused on having a job or career. I was intent on being a wife and a mother. It's true that my husband and I had fights before, and during most of our 14 years I felt he was a cheater—but I deep down I believed he really loved our sons and me.

Most of our married life I had a vague feeling of insecurity to the point that I was taking occasional classes toward my nursing degree, but there was no sense of real urgency. Basically, I often felt like I was used as a doormat, but I hung in there because I really loved him and wanted to keep our family intact.

As a young adult, I remember looking down my Yellow Brick Road and envisioning the many goals I'd set based on the desire to help others. My passion was to delve into the field of nursing, and I visualized how wonderful it would be to work in an environment with like-minded individuals whose primary focus was to help and comfort others.

With my husband's announcement, my Yellow Brick Road plunged me into a muddy hole, stretched wide, with jagged rocks at the bottom and sides so steep I wondered how I would ever get out.

During many sleepless nights, I wondered if my road had ended. I would lie down to sleep in the hole and turn everything over to whatever higher power was out there, my mind swirling until I was exhausted.

Then, as if the Good Witch of the South had landed on my doorstep, miracles started happening. I would awaken in the morning and watch miracle after miracle occur that slowly got me out of the hole. With the heart, courage, and insight of many friends and helpers along the way, my hole grew shallower until I could climb out by myself.

Never more would I be anyone's stupid doormat. I wouldn't be humiliated, lied to, or cheated on any more. I would take my pride and my sons and never be in that kind of situation again.

I felt like Dorothy in the "Wizard of Oz," and, "No Place Like Home" represented me finishing my nursing degree, which would provide security and a happy home. I was motivated to become a nurse at any cost. California had junior colleges, which were cheaper than the colleges in Utah.

One night while sitting in our small condo in California (we had lost our big, beautiful house by now) there was a knock on my front door. I opened it to find a clergyman from the church I belonged to. "Hi," he said. "May I come in?"

Even though it was dark outside and I was a little confused about why he would be at my home so late, I let him in.

"I want to talk to you and your sons," he said.

So I called all my sons into the front room and we gathered around this kind man. Once we were all seated, he said, "I'm not asking, I'm telling you that the Church is going to take care of you."

Astonished, I asked, "What do you mean?"

"We don't want you to go to nursing school now," the clergyman said. "We want you to stay home with your boys."

I wasn't familiar with taking handouts, so I got a little sarcastic when I answered, "Oh, sure. You don't know how many bills we have."

But he was sincere. Even when I showed him my bills, he felt like I could do more good spending time with my boys at this critical time in their lives than by leaving them to get a nursing degree. Having our basic needs taken care of by the church for a year and a half was one of the most humbling experiences in my life. The first time I walked into the church's food warehouse, my eyes filled with tears. It was hard to control myself. After that, I made sure to take one son with me at a time to the warehouse to choose our groceries so they would always remember how God and the Church took care of us.

While I appreciated the time to help my sons adjust to our new reality, my self-esteem was lower than a snake. I kept wondering when my Prince Charming would come along to take care of us and set a good example for my boys. At times I was tempted to go astray and simply allow some nice gentleman to sweep me away, regardless of his core beliefs, but I resisted and hung in there.

My clergyman was very wise because my sons

went crazy and started rebelling, skipping school, and acting out. I had to go to Tough Love Support Group every Thursday night for two years to help raise those boys by myself. It was like building a bridge to make up for the loss of their father. Board by board, nail by nail, I tried to be there for my sons in the way they needed me.

One Christmas we had no money. None. We had food and our bills paid by the Church, but there was no money given to us, so I made each one of my sons a quilt with fabric I already had. We made ornaments to hang on the tiniest Christmas tree that fit in our tiny condo.

On Christmas morning, my ex-husband came and picked up the boys and I was left alone in a condo. I had no relatives in California. I was crushingly lonely, and just wanted to die, but I managed to drag myself to my car and drive to a friend's house. I asked her if I could just sit on a chair in her kitchen for a few minutes. I think dying would have been easier.

Before long, I met a man in my Church who had lost his wife in a car accident a year after my husband left. Still struggling with unbelievable loneliness, I started dating him. He was very kind, especially compared to my past experiences with men. He had a good reputation and appeared to have all the security I needed. The problem was that he had four grieving children who were made up of three teenagers and a seven-year-old. They didn't want their dad dating anyone. Later, I found out they'd made a pledge among themselves that they would never accept me.

After dating for about a year, we thought marriage would work out for us. We got along well, we both belonged to the same religion, and dating him was like good medicine to my emotional wounds. I felt in my heart that God had sent him to me as a miracle. My boys and I would have a roof over our heads, and the Church wouldn't have to take care of us any longer.

So we married, and that's when the trouble really started. In spite of people telling me it would get better and the children would adjust, things just got worse and worse. We all went to group therapy once a week, but the children wouldn't speak to each other. It was like having the Continental Divide in our house. We tried everything, but it just wasn't working.

The Yellow "Sick" Road

I started having panic attacks. Many nights I would wake up in sweat, shaking uncontrollably. I would go down to the sofa or out on the front lawn just to catch my breath. I felt like I was suffocating, and wondered if I was going insane.

Finally, after not doing anything for months but resting beside a fireplace and watching movies, I started to get better. I enrolled in nursing school, which empowered me. If I could just finish my nursing degree, I could take care of my sons myself and get out of this dysfunctional marriage. My husband stated that he knew I had done everything I could to get along with his children, and he didn't blame me for leaving. I stayed in the relationship for 12 years, and he and I remain friends.

While driving in the old silver station wagon, my sons and I would sometimes sing:

> Oh, we don't have a barrel of money
> Maybe we're ragged and funny
> But we're traveling along
> Singing a song
> Side by side.
> Through all kinds of weather

Cyclone

Whether the sky shall fall
Just as long as we're together
It really doesn't matter at all.

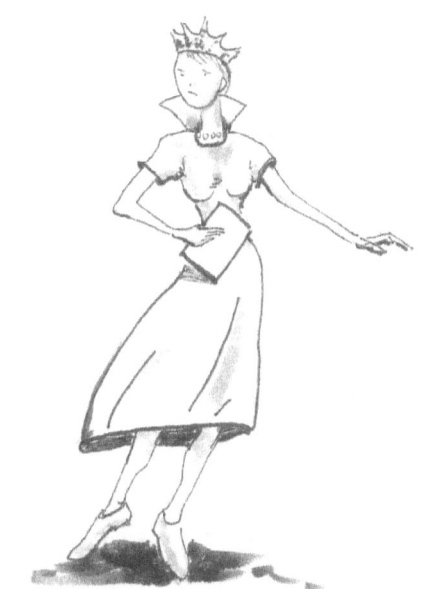

Chapter Two: Flash Cards

Nothing in my life has ever been easy. I grew up accustomed to work. When I was a little girl, my dad paid me a nickel to sweep out the garage. I would sing at neighbors' houses and they would give me a few coins that I would spend on penny candy. One lady gave me an old brown banana. It was awful looking and I just threw it away. Maybe she didn't like the song I sang. The song went like this:

Flash Cards

My mom gave me a nickel to buy a pickle
I didn't buy a pickle,
I got some chewing gum
Chew, chew, chew, chew, chew, gum
I bought some chewing gum
To chew, chew, chew

I was still trying to raise my own children and stepchildren while finishing nursing school, and it was sooo hard. Many times I felt guilty and wondered if I was taking too much time away from my children, who were always my priority. Many times I took my bag of nursing flash cards to soccer games and events the children were in and studied while trying to support their many activities. During all this time, my stepchildren hated me and were being vindictive and hatefully rebellious.

Sometimes in the middle of the night I'd drive up to the college and look in the glass case to see if my grade was posted. In order to stay in the program, we had to have a "B" average and couldn't get anything lower than a "C."

School has always been hard for me. I was never

The Yellow "Sick" Road

the kind of student who could just read something to memorize it and then go take a test. As the Jr. Class Secretary in my high school, I had to maintain a certain grade point average. It was a challenge for me to keep my grades up in order to stay in different school organizations. It was hard juggling grades and social life.

After utilizing tutors, flash cards by the hundreds in little baggies, lectures taped on my little old-fashioned cassette tape recorder, studying, and taking tests—I finally graduated with an Associate's Degree in Nursing.

My third son, Scott, was in a lot of activities, including being named Prom king and becoming a local football star as well as a wrestling star. He had so much enthusiasm and love for life that his football team members called him, "the motivator." Everybody knew him, and he was so well loved that he's probably still a legend in the town.

At 21 years old, he was on his way to Idaho with his high school girlfriend to attend college. I was sitting on the beach after working a long night shift when one of my other sons came running to me, yelling, "Mom! Mom! Come to the phone, quick! It's

Scott! He's been in a car accident and his hand… something about his hand!"

I jumped up and ran to the pay phone where a police officer told me that Scott was in a tiny hospital in Del, Montana. I frantically called the hospital and learned that Scott was in a coma and his hand was almost severed from his arm. He'd fallen asleep at the wheel while driving over a bridge at 10 a.m. In the crash, he was ejected from the car, but his girlfriend had her seat belt on and wasn't so severely injured.

When I spoke to his girlfriend, she said they'd had to use the paddles twice. I knew what that meant. His heart had stopped twice, and they were trying to shock it back to life.

In a daze, I managed to take the next flight out from Orange County Airport in California to the Salt Lake City University Hospital, where Scott was being transferred. By the time I arrived, the paramedics had just brought him into the ER (emergency room.)

It was difficult to face his injuries alone, but I tried to hold myself together. I tried explaining to the nurses that I was a nurse and wanted to see my son right now. They made me wait, which nearly turned me into one of those hysterical family members that a nurse doesn't ever want to deal with.

Finally, they let me see Scott. They had intubated him and his hand was elevated high above his head. I stared at him in disbelief, and then cried out, "Is there an Elder in the hospital to give him a blessing?" (In my church, an Elder is like a pastor.)

Suddenly, there were two of the most innocent looking young men ready to give a healing blessing.

I stayed with Scott for a solid month. At one time, I lay on a sofa in the foyer and cried for about two hours. Suddenly, a lady approached and offered to stay with me. I asked her who she was.

"A doctor's wife," she replied.

I will never forget the comfort she gave me. Since that time of such personal emotional devastation, I am extra sensitive to people in distress. Like the Tin Man in Oz who wanted a heart, I have a heart full of caring for all humanity, and want to give back some of what this kindly woman freely offered me.

It is difficult to be a nurse to your own son. Scott recovered somewhat, and kept his hand, but he continuously deal with the after effects of TBI (Traumatic Brain Injury). Not only did he have to learn to walk and talk all over again, but has suffered emotionally with anger and loss. He lost his girlfriend, his identity, and his ability to keep a job because of his problem with impulsivity. He is currently living on disability.

Although my Yellow Brick Road had taken another unexpected turn, I felt as if passing my Boards of Nursing was the answer to all my problems. I was sure that now I could get control of my life. I was on my way.

Little did I know I was going to start another road—a road I call The Yellow Sick Road of nursing.

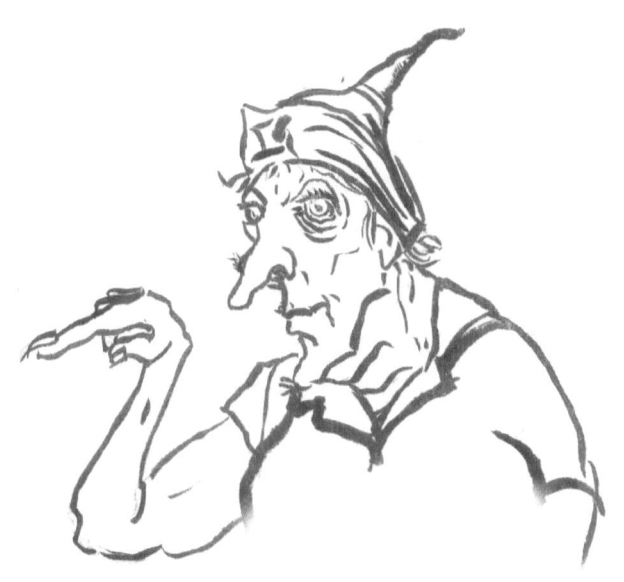

Chapter Three: Knobby Finger

After graduating from nursing school in 1991, I worked mainly in acute rehab at several large California hospitals. After a time, I felt the desire to move back to Utah. My sister had just bought a historic pioneer home in the southern part of Utah for $27,000.00. Her purchase piqued my curiosity, so I took a few days off to fly to Utah to see if I could find a pioneer home for myself.

It was so refreshing to get out of California and

escape to this quiet place that I met with a real estate agent. I told her I had four hours to buy a pioneer home. After looking at two, I decided on one that was near a hospital, and began the process of purchasing it. I put it on my credit card, with the intent of moving back to Utah to start a new life.

I used to sing John Denver's "Country Roads" as I drove from California to my little pioneer house. I was going to start over and try and save myself. I wanted to bring my wild surfing sons to Utah to get away from the California environment, so I rented a U-Haul trailer to move all our stuff, and off we went.

My old pioneer home was such a sanctuary that I drove back and forth from California to Utah for several years as I tried to get stability in my life.

Single again, I would sometimes work an all-night shift, then drive all day to get to my pioneer home. I felt so secure in my rural home with a hospital close by, where I worked from time to time while making the transition. I wanted to stay there permanently.

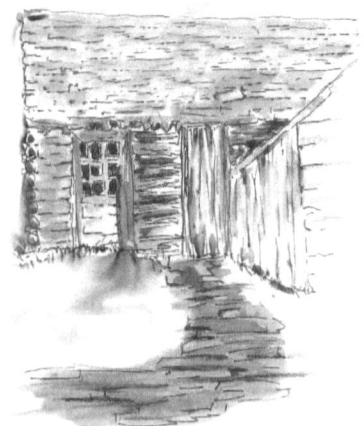

The Yellow "Sick" Road

It seemed as if miracles happened when the director of nursing at the rural hospital encouraged me to work there. I felt such love and warmth from her that I wondered how my life could be so good. I was traveling a pleasant stretch of the Yellow Brick Road.

To clarify what rural hospital is, it is a hospital that is very consolidated. This means that nurses must overlap their responsibilities by doing med/ surg/tele, (medical/surgical/telemetry-or cardiac)- labor and delivery, and ER. It is one of the most difficult nursing jobs there is because you have to be able to do all of these units proficiently.

I was getting more confident in my nursing skills when I started working at the rural hospital. However, the complete move was made over a period of one and a half years, which made it necessary to work in both California and Utah. It was a long, thought out decision. There was no place like my pioneer home, which offered a sanctuary to get away from all the family problems, heartache, and confusion in my California environment. My emotional state of mind was near to its breaking point, so it was either make a decision and move on, or get swept up in the twisted swirl of California life.

With just one more load of belongings to move into my new sanctuary, I was hired full time at the local hospital and began to feel at ease. The people appeared to be kind and laid back; the kind of people who could easily become friends.

As I pulled up to my house with my final load of stuff in a U-Haul, I heard the phone ringing. I ran in to answer it and found myself speaking to the Director of Nursing (DON), who asked to see me. We met in her office.

What unfolded was a reprimand that hit me like a ton of bricks. She pointed at a paper where she'd written a whole list of things I needed to improve in my work. In short, I was on probation. The experience left me shocked, speechless and numb. She may as well have been the Wicked Witch of the West, long green nose, warts and all as I focused on her knobby finger pointing at the paper before shaking that same witchlike finger at me.

There was nothing very specific on her list, and nothing major that would cause serious

The Yellow "Sick" Road

problems or put any patient at risk. I sat there, horrified, because I had just made the final move to Utah and had the impression I was doing fine, and now I was on probation.

Finally, at the end of her "shape up or ship out" speech, I pulled myself out of a shocked stupor and told her I had never been called in and reprimanded in such a manner before. I asked why she hadn't told me earlier that she was not satisfied with my work. She just looked at me. Then I informed her that I would let her know the next day what I would do.

My world seemed to crumble as I went home. In my two years of nursing, I had only been called in once, and that was about missing a minor medication at a California hospital.

I couldn't sleep all night. I just lay there, frozen to the bed, all manner of thoughts running through my mind. I felt betrayed by fellow employees who I thought of as friends. In my mind, I pictured them backbiting and gossiping about me. I had trusted them. They knew of the personal tragedies I had been going through. I felt like I had been set up, with no warning or compassion.

The next day I got up, dressed, and made a

phone call to meet with the DON. I drew all the courage I could muster and told her that I was not going to work there any longer due to the environment of hypocrisy and double standards. I went on to say that I did not respect her or the other nurses, people I initially thought were up front and honest. I asked her why I wasn't advised that my work performance had been perceived as poor before I moved everything from California. Again, she didn't answer me.

So I said, "I will never set foot in this place again."

Her reply was, "If you do that, you can never be re-hired."

I told her it didn't matter, because I didn't wish to work with people like them.

If there was ever a Wicked Witch of the West, it was this lady. Her calculating manner was uncaring, detached, and lacked compassion. In her lecture to me, her voice was raspy, which made her sound as if she were cackling when she raised her voice in a scolding manner, making it clear in no uncertain terms that I was beneath her.

I was so upset that I called my bishop (a religious pastor in my church) because he was also one of the doctors on the hospital board. I told him what happened, and described her manner of dealing with me. "She professes to be so religious, but she sure wasn't very Christlike in that meeting," I said. "Will you please inform the hospital board of her actions?"

He said there was nothing he could do to change what had happened.

I told him that I wasn't asking for my job back, I just want the incident reported.

He agreed, and reported it for me.

For the next few months I drove back to my old job, living out of motels, paying thousands of dollars for gas and expenses to work in the state of California again.

Then a nurse in my neighborhood who'd heard what happened told me about a job at a psychiatric hospital in Salt Lake City. Even with the high honors he received in the naval academy the rural hospital still fired him, leaving his family destitute, so he had some idea of how I felt.

Knobby Finger

I followed his recommendation, and thankfully, I got the job.

This was the beginning of my encounters with abusive nurses who have no compassion for staff. This is why those who work in management need to go through personality testing to see if they are a good fit for the job, and then go through training to learn the required professionalism of working in the nursing field. How could a DON be nice to patients if she can't be nice to her staff?

No matter the age or job title, a bully always does harm.

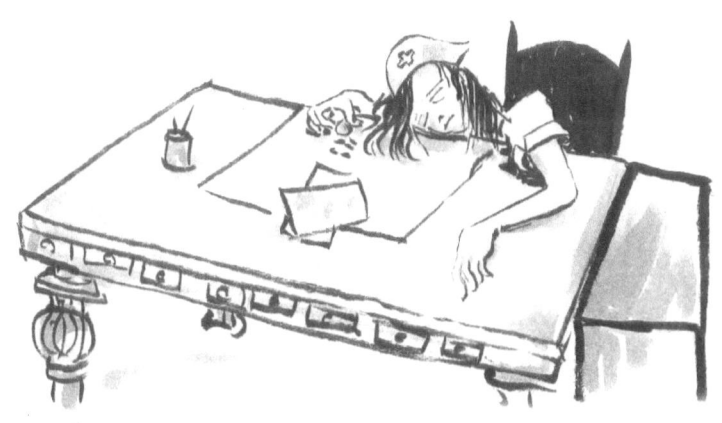

Chapter Four:
The Witch's Spell

After working in the mental hospital for six months, I felt it just wasn't for me. I appreciated the nurse who'd stuck his neck out to help me get the job, because it seems as though most nurses are scared to death to speak up for one another. I will always remember him helping me, and pray that his life has been blessed for his efforts.

I was still trying to get over what had happened to me in the rural hospital when I came across a newspaper ad for a Director of Nursing job in a care center in Salt Lake City. I had never been in management before, but I was interested in learning more about it, so I applied. I was excited when I was offered the job. This would be a different challenge for me, and I was all for it, highly motivated to discover what a good leader is made of in the world of nursing.

I learned about hiring and firing, coding, billing, policies and procedures, laws, privacy, etc. Anything you can name pertaining to nursing, I had to learn. In spite of the rigorous training, I really enjoyed this exciting new challenge. Even after working as Director of Nursing for six months, I was still learning.

The administrator was very patient with me, but one day he called me into his office to tell me that while they really liked me, they'd brought in a nurse who had director experience. He asked me to stay on as the Assistant Director of Nursing (ADON). It was a little hard to step down, but I was okay with it, since I still felt I had a lot to learn. I decided I could learn more from the experienced DON.

Little did I know that she had a history of drug

use that was significant enough to earn her a place in the Diversion Program, a probationary state instituted by the Board of Registered Nursing. This meant that she had to submit to spontaneous drug tests in order to be allowed to continue working as a nurse.

Nobody told me she was being monitored for drug use. I had to find that out for myself.

Meanwhile, I was responsible for the narcotic drug count, which meant that I was accountable for all the narcotics that were locked in my office with a double key. Once a month, every narcotic drug had to balance with the accounting of what had been administered.

One evening when the DON was on the Medicare unit, she told a nurse that she would take care of giving morphine to a certain patient for pain. I was a little curious about her offer to do such a routine task, so after she was done, I checked the morphine count and discovered that we were short one.

This made me so nervous that I went to the administrator's office and reported it. He said he would check into it. That's when he admitted to me that this DON was on the Diversion Program because

The Witch's Spell

of her history of drug use.

All of a sudden it made sense to me as to why she always seemed so sedated at our morning meetings. As if under a witch's spell in "The Wizard of Oz's" sleep-inducing poppy fields, she could hardly keep her eyes open. Her behavior began adding up, and I realized that I was working under the direction of a drug user. This was crazy. I really liked my job, but how was this going to work out with her stealing drugs?

The administrator didn't seem to do much about the situation. He acted as though the only thing that mattered was that she knew how to do Medicare coding, scheduling, etc. I heard that he had a history of using pot, so I was most likely trying to deal with an enabler.

After I reported the missing morphine to the administrator, the DON looked for ways to sabotage me. If I was going to tell on her, she obviously wanted me out of there. When she began reporting my "faults" to the administrator, I could see the writing on the wall. I had to get out.

The Yellow "Sick" Road

At this point I'd like to state that there are caring nurses out there as well as competent and caring management personnel, yet those who are incompetent to do the job should not be allowed to practice.

I applied at a Big hospital in Salt Lake City where I hoped I could advance in learning all the exciting things nurses love to do. Once I was hired, I gave the care center notice of my departure. The hardest part of leaving a job is the love felt for the patients and some of the staff. I had been there for two and a half years, and my love for the residents made my day of departure a very sad one, but I knew I couldn't continue working in that environment.

One resident in particular was cute in her own way. Alice had a big personality in her elderly body, proudly displayed a poster of Tom Selleck above her bed, and was very outspoken. In spite of the fact that her room always smelled vaguely of urine because of her indwelling urine catheter, I was drawn to her. She was the president of the Resident's Council, and I miss her endearing, bossy ways to this day.

One night after I began working at the Big hospital, I visited Alice, tip-toeing into her room to say, "Hi." She was surprised to see me, and happy to give me one last hug.

After starting my new job, I heard that the care center DON had been fired. She'd lost her license and was in prison for stealing drugs at the facility. Yep, I knew that's what should have happened when I was there, but nobody followed through with any disciplinary consequences until after I left.

Another crooked spot in the Yellow Sick Road. Is this what nursing is all about?

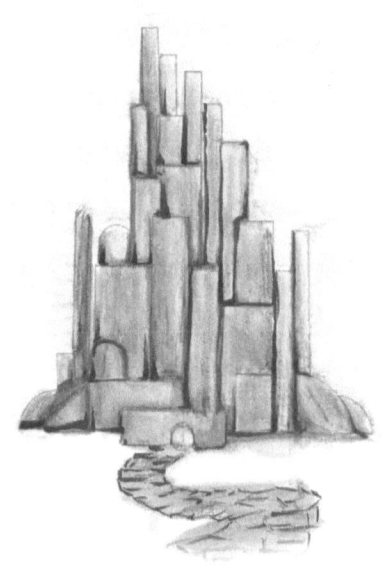

Chapter Five: Emerald City—Illusion

My Imagination Hospital

My new place of employment with its big 300-bed facility appeared to me as full of promise as the Emerald City, a place of limitless possibilities. In order to explain how I relate the Wizard of Oz characters to the positive side of nursing, allow me to say that I hoped this hospital would be such a bright emerald green that I would

Emerald City—Illusion

have to wear sunglasses.

At the gate, a man clothed in green would say, "I am the guardian of the gate." After admittance, I would open the elevator door and find myself in a wonderful place. If not for my dark glasses, the palatial hospital halls would blind me because of their brightness.

This is where I hoped my Yellow Brick Road would take me to new and pleasant learning experiences, where the great, almighty OZ would show me how to obtain the secure feeling of home, sweet home, because there's no place like home. I imagined happily providing all the care a nurse could possibly do in treating the largest wounds and applying healing dressings. Helping my patients feel better and aid their healing would be the greatest life I could imagine.

I already knew I could handle this job without passing out, and I anticipated a fascinating and educational experience in learning more about all the bodily fluids and tissues of the skin. This was a dream come true, where I'd be proud to wear my nursing scrubs. I envisioned other nurses and aides as copartners, with high morale, and everyone working

The Yellow "Sick" Road

with fairly distributed patient loads.

As I enter the unit where I am to work, an extra-large chair serves as a throne for the charge nurse. As I

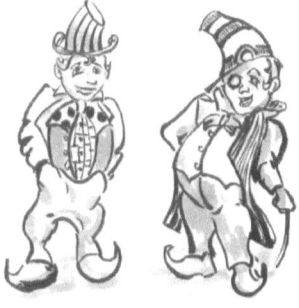

approach her, I would humbly ask her what my assignment was for the day. I gratefully take my little Munchkin patients, thrilled to serve them. It was wonderful to learn and serve at the same time.

I would be given the Winged Monkey assistants to fly around, accessible to help lift and turn the patients before I even had to ask them. They were so swift and fast as to make the nurse's job almost miraculous. It was as though the ruby slippers I wore did the walking for me so that I was not even tired at the end of the day.

I felt certain that the Emerald City would help me feel brave, to develop a warm heart and develop the knowledge in my brain to become an even better nurse. A day at work would bring the echoing voice of the great Oz through the hospital speakers, inviting all the staff to have prayers in order to give thanks and offer blessings to service our wonderful Munchkin patients.

Emerald City—Illusion

In my imagination, the gardens were full of orange colored poppies at lunchtime, the sedating fragrance aiding in relaxation. The garden of poppies, accompanied by little waterfalls and quaint little birds, erased all anxiety. Food delivered by the Flying Monkeys matched the scenery and your tastes, delivered faster than I could lift a magic wand.

Again, the great Oz would speak after lunch, asking how the food was, and if there was anything he could do to make it better. He would be there to help the staff have a great day.

I would walk back through the palace halls and the elevator would swish me up to my unit to take care of the patients. The charge nurse was on her throne with her magic wand while all the other nurses smiled and networked in order to help one another.

The charge nurses were the Good Witches of the South and North, and wore the most beautiful flowing pink scrub gowns. They had the kindest, most gentle faces, and their wisdom and knowledge surrounded them. When I approached, they would receive me with acceptance and love abounding. There was never hesitancy in asking them a question. They would all but beg me to help me solve any problem that should arise. I felt like the perfect nurse with the brains, heart, and courage to take care of my patients with the best of medical care.

The patients' wounds and illnesses healed rapidly because of the great love surrounding them. Their families were pleased and hopeful in seeing their loved ones getting better because the aides were so in tune to their needs. The family members would be so appreciative of us helping to heal the patients they would bring us exquisite food, including grapes and apples.

I could hardly wait to go to work. Just being around all the staff made it a place you hated to leave. There was no place like the Emerald City Hospital.

When Friday's payday came, I would stand in line, waiting for my gold coins to be weighed on a scale. While I waited, the Wizard of Oz would sing "Somewhere Over the Rainbow" over the intercom. We would all get an extra coin just for coming in to pick up our pay. The head nurses would use their magic wands and touch our foreheads with gratitude for our service. If we had any aliments from our hard work, they would be taken away with the explanation that it was the least they could do for all our hard work.

Nursing would be worth all of the cyclone years of study and raising my children as a single parent. It would be worth marrying husband #2 and taking care of four stepchildren for 12 years. There wasn't anything more wonderful than being a nurse in the Emerald City Hospital.

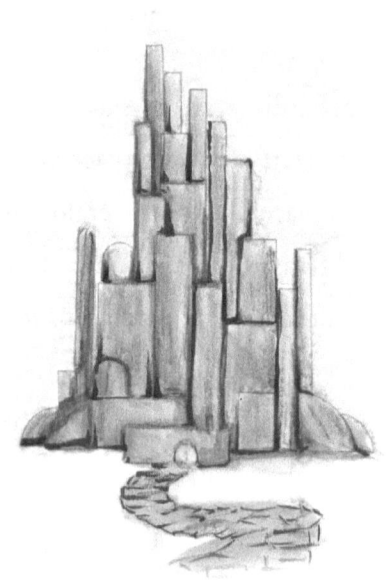

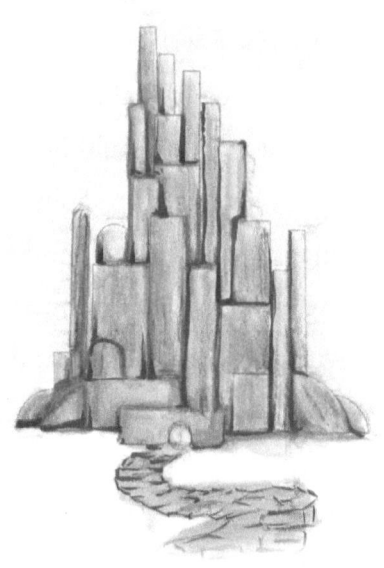

Chapter Six: Emerald City—Real

"I've a feeling we're not in Kansas anymore."

But, unfortunately I had to wake up to reality. My dream was all an illusion. My Yellow Sick Road was crooked and lined with ditches full of mud – yet again, sometimes there were pleasant, happy times in caring for my patients.

The nurse/patient assignments that are given for

the day are crucial. As I walked onto the unit and looked at the board to see how the charge nurse had distributed the patient load, it would be like watching either a floating or a sinking ship. Some nurses even came in early and change the assignment board so they had the easy patients. Management usually let them get away with it because they were their friends. I decided I would rather tolerate their re-assignment than complain because it usually didn't do any good to speak up about it. The charge nurse would usually just be defensive.

I doubt very much if the general public even has a clue what the nurse on the shift may be going through. If the assignments are unfair, the patient is the one that suffers most, especially when there are emergency needs. If harm takes place to a patient assigned to a nurse, the nurse is held responsible and can get written up.

An example of a really dangerous and dysfunctional assignment at the Big hospital is when I came to work on a night shift and the charge nurse gave herself two patients and gave me seven. Needless to say, I was scared and

The Yellow "Sick" Road

overwhelmed. When I asked the charge nurse about it, she just ignored me.

This particular charge nurse's reputation was such that she would try to get out of work while the rest of the staff ran around like crazy, trying to take care of all the patients and answer their call lights. Management knew this about her, but didn't do anything about it.

Still, for the protection of my patients and my nurse license, I called the supervisor and informed her about the dangerous, overloaded assignment. The supervisor came, investigated the situation, and took one patient away from me and gave it back to the charge nurse.

Most of the time a night nurse would have only six patients at the most, yet I have watched charge nurses dump on nurses time after time while sitting at their desks, heads propped up, trying to prevent themselves from falling asleep.

Sometimes I've been tempted to accidentally/on purpose bump into the chair of a dozing charge nurse to see if she might fall to the floor. That would be real interesting for her if she fell off the chair and broke her arm. She'd have to do an incident report and make a worker's compensation claim. I guess she would have to write down on the form that she had fallen asleep on her chair.

In the real world, a nurse would have severe consequences for sleeping on the job. Some facilities would fire you on the spot if you went to sleep, even on your break or lunch.

When I realized what I was thinking, my thoughts sounded like complaining nurses—ones I never wanted to be like. Yet my night shifts were like nightmares. Rarely did I feel like I had met all the needs of my patients. Most of the nurses never felt any satisfaction or reward after their shift because they were too overwhelmed. Some days after working all night, I couldn't sleep because I would think of things that probably should have been done, and my mind would swim with worry.

The term "aide" was a joke, because they didn't seem to be around when needed. I would have to look all around for the aides when I needed help. They were not like the Flying Monkeys in my Emerald City Illusion who were there before you even asked

The Yellow "Sick" Road

for their help.

In reality, they were flying, all right –flying away so that you couldn't find them.

I once got so desperate for an aide's help that when my dog had puppies, I gave one to her, because it was a particular breed of puppy that she'd always wanted. I thought that if I gave it to her, she would feel an obligation to help me on the job.

But it didn't make a difference. I still had to beg her for help and repeatedly had to explain why I needed her assistance. "Please help me turn this patient," I'd plead, "please help me toilet her."

The aides often just visited and joked with the charge nurse or management, then goofed off and went into hiding, sometimes even to the point of leaving the hospital and going out to the parking lot. It was against hospital policy to leave the hospital without clocking out or without permission.

Another nurse reported to me that she had informed management that the aides were dealing drugs outside. It was supposedly being investigated, but I didn't ever see consequences of any type.

Poor management, favoritism, unfair and dangerous patient assignments, and missing aides are just a few examples of what was going on in this Big hospital.

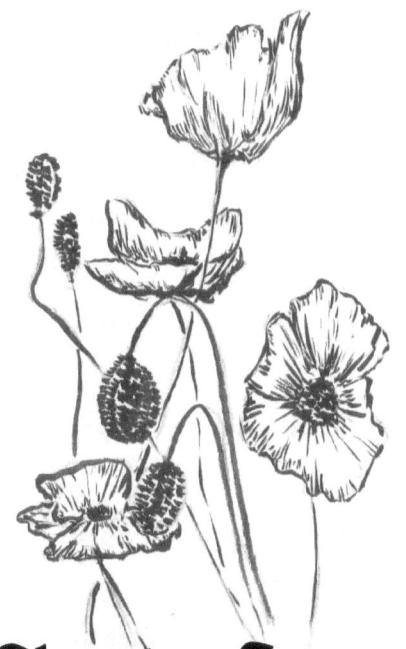

Chapter Seven: Dead Daughter

Sad, Sad, Story

This chapter doesn't necessarily deal with the dysfunction of the Big hospital, but is one of the saddest experiences I went through as a nurse. We nurses are human and emotional and have trauma situations that we never forget.

A patient in her forties was admitted for multiple diagnoses, including high blood sugar. When she was

Dead Daughter

assigned to me, we got along right off the bat, even though she had a reputation as a "frequent flier," which refers to a patient who tries to be admitted with complaints of pain sufficient to get narcotics. I could tell she felt as comfortable around me as I did with her.

I had just done her admit paper work when the charge nurse pulled me aside to tell me that the woman's 19-year-old daughter was dead in the ER from an apparent drug overdose.

I asked the charge nurse what we should do. We brainstormed and decided to call pastoral care first to see if a clergyman would tell the patient about her daughter. When he arrived, he agreed it was the best way to inform the patient of her loss. The hospital pastors are trained for this type of grieving and traumatic situation. When the pastor went into the woman's room, my heart sank. I was very emotional and upset. I wanted to run, and then again, I wanted to stay and comfort the mother.

Suddenly, a bellowing scream come out of the room. It was loud and ongoing, resounding throughout the whole hospital. After a while, it became a sob that wouldn't quit.

The Yellow "Sick" Road

Finally, I had to go in the room to administer some medication that was due. As I walked in, I saw that the mother's face appeared flat and lifeless. She sat in her bed, hardly moving.

When I walked up to her I said, "I'm so sorry."

The pastor had encouraged the patient to see her daughter's body. He said it was necessary for her to accept the death and move forward with the grieving process. I was supportive of the pastor's professional advice.

After spending some time with my patient, I asked if she wanted to go down and see her daughter. She replied, "NO, NO!"

Finally, after some gentle persuasion, she said she would go if I went with her. I took a big breath and agreed.

She got in a wheelchair and I pushed her along the halls, my feet moving slowly. I needed to be there for my patient, but I kept wondering how I was going to hold up while trying to be strong for this mother.

We got on the elevator and went down to what felt to me like the tunnel of doom. I didn't know what to expect when we reached the daughter's body. To this day, my recollections of that event are overshadowed by a kind of blankness. I just remember this mother saying over and over, "Is that you? Is that you?" She didn't touch her daughter much. She mainly sat in her wheelchair and cried. I kept reminding myself that the pastor had said this would be very painful for the mother, but would help her to accept her daughter's death and aid her grieving in the future.

When she was done, I slowly rolled the patient back to the elevator and up to her room. Deep down I just wanted to go home, shut myself in my own room, and cry. I wanted to cry for my patient and cry because it also reminded me of how I would feel if I had lost one of my own children. I gave a sigh of relief that I still had my four sons—in spite of all the problems they'd had, not only with Scott's accident, but also from their dad leaving and the effects of two divorces.

This was a dark day on the Yellow Sick Road.

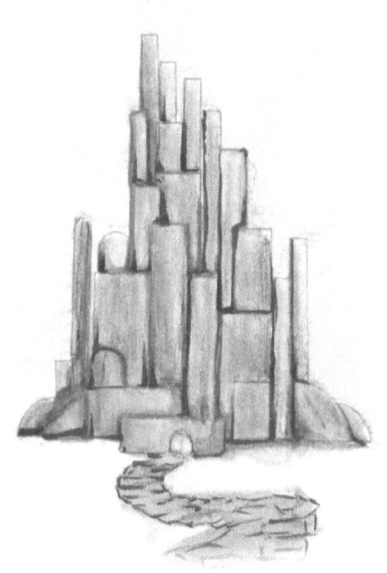

Chapter Eight: Emerald City—Falling

"Thanks, George."

There was a nurse I'll call George who was at the Big hospital where I worked for 7 years. One day, George suddenly began yelling at me in the hallway. He was full blown yelling in front of all the patients and staff. He caught me off guard, and I couldn't really understand what he was saying.

Finally, I asked him to please come into the lounge where I hoped he'd settle down so I could understand what was going on. Eventually, it came out that George blamed me for making a female nurse friend of his cry. Apparently, he got word that I had mentioned to another male nurse that I was tired of two nurses who would go off to lunch together for over an hour when we were only allowed half hour lunches. While they were gone for so long, the other nurses had to take care of the two nurse's patients. I only mentioned this to the other nurse because he was on duty, and I wondered how he was doing with the task of taking care of his own patients as well as those assigned to the other two nurses.

He didn't say much to me, but let the two nurses know I'd been complaining about their absence, which made one of them cry. Now George was giving me an earful for what I'd said.

Well, I'm sorry my words made the nurse cry, but there would be a lot more crying if something happened to the patients because they weren't getting the care they needed from short staffing. It was all so stupid and blown out of perspective that it was ridiculous. The encounter left me shaking.

The Yellow "Sick" Road

I went into the manager's office to let her know of this abusive behavior. She acted like it was no big deal, which wasn't surprising since she had shown favoritism toward George. Still, she said she'd take care of it.

I don't know whether it was ever taken care of, but George never acted any different to me one way or the other. He continued to do just about whatever he wanted, and apparently getting away with it.

There were a lot of politics at the Big hospital. After I'd been there for seven years, I worried about making enough money for retirement, so when a nurse friend of mine said there was a good job opportunity working travel nurse contracts, I listened. She mentioned an opportunity in a little rural medicine hospital in Nevada.

After I interviewed for the travel nurse job, it was offered to me. I gave notice at the Big hospital, but I stayed per diem. That meant that I was still considered an employee and would only need to work on the schedule three days a month to keep that status. It sounded good to me because I still planned to retire from the Big hospital to take advantage of the excellent retirement and medical benefits package.

The travel assignment worked out well. My contract was extended multiple times, allowing me to work for them for a year. This added income allowed me to pay off my debts.

I was now ready to go back to the Big hospital, but thought it might be a better idea to transfer to a sister hospital that was only 50 minute drive from my pioneer house. So I interviewed at the hospital and got the job. Since it was a sister hospital, my retirement and benefits package was intact. I was so excited at the idea of finishing up my old age years with good medical benefits and retirement.

It was so important to me to have things work out well at this hospital that I decided to see a counselor that I could talk things over with so that I wouldn't blow it. I found a very reputable counselor with a medical background and a doctorate degree. I was very open to everything he talked about, and receptive to any advice he had to offer.

I was so hopeful and optimistic on my first day at working in the hospital that when they said, "Jump" I jumped. Unfortunately, I overheard that this hospital was having a lot of problems regarding firing employees for some pretty minor offenses. This usually meant that they were micromanaging everything.

After I'd worked there for a month, I was written up for not labeling a lab vial correctly. Even though I told the manager I'd done it the way my training nurse had shown me, it didn't seem to make any difference. She proceeded to inform me that three offenses would result in my automatic termination, which made it seem as if the manager would be watching my every move from now on. I felt like I was being blackballed already.

I mentioned the incident to my counselor, who recommended that I document everything.

On another occasion, I was asked to float (transfer to another floor) to do pediatric patients. I was willing to do it, but stated that even though I knew a little about it, I had not been hired to work in pediatrics.

The departing nurse let me know that one of my patients was the 12-year-old daughter of a doctor on staff. This patient had lesions in her nose and throat that made it very difficult for her to eat. The nurse informed me that the girl's father was not authorized to write orders for his own daughter. If he did, I was to call the manager.

As soon as the nurse left, the doctor came in and started writing orders for his daughter to have an NG (neogastric) tube put down her nose so she could have liquid feedings.

Following the departing nurse's instructions, I called the manager. She asked to talk to the doctor. Once he was on the phone, he yelled at her. Then he turned on me and said he would have both our jobs. I refused to help him with a procedure called "conscious sedation" as it was out of my scope of practice. He got more furious at me by the minute.

The charge nurse ended up calling a nurse from the ER to come and help him with the procedure.

It appears that after I told the supervisor what had happened, it went clear to the top, coming to the attention of the director of nursing. The next day, I was called into the manager's office. She offered me no support at all for my actions in following the departing nurse's directives, but instead informed me that she'd begun a file on me. So instead of management appreciating me following procedure, they turned on me.

The Yellow "Sick" Road

This experience taught me that in many instances, a doctor is always right, no matter what. The hospital wants their patients, and the patients go where their doctor refers them. The hospital does not want to get on a doctor's bad side, because then he or she will not send patients their way, and that was what was important to the hospital—the mighty dollar.

After this incident, I noticed my shifts were scheduled for only a few days. If I put myself down as being available for an extra shift, I wouldn't get it. Even though staff nurses were supposed to have priority, the manager would give the shift I requested to some per diem nurse. She defended her actions by saying that she could give shifts to anybody she wanted to.

In my mind, I felt like I was in a dark forest where the air was starting to smother me.

One night, management called me in just before my night shift began to address the complaint of an aide who'd reported that I should have called a "Rapid Response" on a patient who was having breathing problems. When I'd assessed the patient, his breathing was a normal pattern for him, and he was stable. I also had the charge nurse assess him, and we were both in agreement that he was stable. But the aide thought she knew more than the nurses. In spite of the charge nurse's concurring evaluation, I was written up from an aide's assessment of my patient.

This particular aide was a personal friend of manager's, and would sleep half the night when she was supposed to be working. When I mentioned her behavior to the manager, she said she was aware of it and that it was ok because the woman had children to take care of in the morning.

Good grief—how would the family members feel if they knew they were paying an aide to sleep?

Everything seemed to be backfiring. As I sat in a monthly nurse meeting, I listened to the HR (human resources) man say, "Now if any of you have any problems, please just come to me." I really believed this man to be sincerely on my side. He was a man of good standing in a church he belonged to, and appeared to be someone I could trust. So, in

The Yellow "Sick" Road

confidence and almost in tears, I talked to him after the meeting.

That turned on me, too. Pretty soon I got called in with the DON, management, and some people who made up a panel of ancillary employees. When they interrogated me, I knew I was doomed. The HR guy turned out to be like a little spy, and now I realized that his job was to find out any dissenters and then get them out of the hospital.

To top it off, one snowy, stormy night after working the night shift, I drove home so exhausted that I was simply happy I hadn't slid off the icy road and crashed.

As I walked into my home, tired and looking forward to plopping into my bed, the phone rang. It was my manager telling me that I had to come back and sign an order the doctor had written to have a patient discharged.

By now I had worked in management as well as a DON, so I knew there was no real urgency to sign the order that night. A kind manager would just hold it and allow me to sign it when I came in for my next shift. So I asked her, "Can't I just sign it when I come in again on my next shift?"

"No."

So with eyes blurry from fatigue and suffering such emotional pain that this manager would insist on this unnecessary trip through dangerous driving conditions, I'm surprised I didn't crash. It took over an hour to get back to the hospital and two seconds to sign the order. This act of harassment proved to me that she was trying to run me out. I could see the writing on the wall.

In a panic, I decided I would try to go back to working at the Big hospital where I had left in good standing. All I really wanted was a simple transfer. When I talked to my former manager and asked for an interview to get my old job back, she said she was sorry but there were no openings at this time. I believed her because I didn't see any jobs posted for that unit.

Yet there were other openings on another unit, and I felt very confident that I could get a job there. To be sure of doing my best, I watched interviewing videos and studied which things to do and not do. At last, I dressed in my best and went to the interview. My hands were sweating and my nerves were making me shake.

The Yellow "Sick" Road

What happened next has probably never happened to anybody else on this earth. As I was in the interview, answering the unit manager's questions, a big voice boomed, "DON'T HIRE CLAUDIA SANBORN." Both the interviewer and myself were shocked into silence. It turned out that the manager was wearing what is called a "vocera" around his neck, a device that makes it easy to instantly contact people throughout the hospital. He'd forgotten to turn it off during the interview.

We both looked at each other. He was as embarrassed as I was. I asked if he wanted to continue with the interview. I did my best to finish answering his questions, but it was next to impossible.

Stumbling towards the elevator, I got on and rode down to the HR office. I told them what happened, and they replied that they didn't know anything about it.

When I got back into the elevator, the aide I had given a puppy to years earlier was there. She hinted that something was going on, and whispered for me to call her. She had always been one who knew everybody's business, but I was so numb and so focused on reaching my car and getting away that I didn't even get her phone number. In my heart, I think it was George who had sabotaged me. He probably knew I was interviewing and didn't want me to come back.

I thought about calling an attorney about the situation, but I was afraid to pursue it. I'd heard from a hotline that dealt with bullying in the workforce that you shouldn't try to sue your employer because you don't have a chance. Even if by some miracle you win the case, you'd be blackballed and never get a nursing job anywhere ever again.

Years later, as I worked toward retirement, I talked to several attorneys who said they would have taken the case in a minute, but the statute of limitations had passed, so there was nothing they could do now.

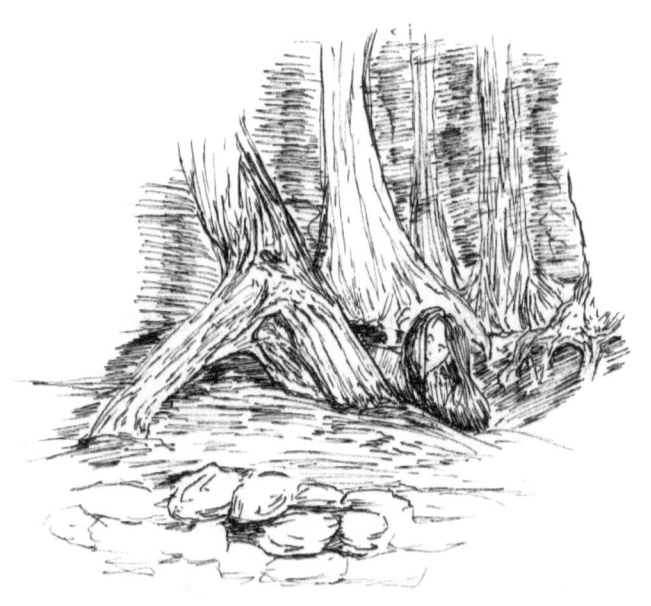

Chapter Nine: The Ditch

Have you ever been in a ditch? I'm talking about a muddy, slimy hole.

When I was in this metaphorical ditch, I was desperate to find a way out. As I waddled through the muck, I finally found a big root sticking out of the oozing mud near the top of the ditch. I grabbed it, and with all my strength, pulled myself out.

This is what I felt like after enduring the

The Ditch

disastrous interview and all the prior incidents in the rural sister hospital. I knew what was coming next—a hospital wide layoff—which would ruin my plan for retirement. I was too old to be hired at any hospital. They'd most likely just look at me and say, "Honey, you need to retire, not be hired."

Then the dreaded phone call came. The hospital wanted me to come in at 3:00 the next day.

I couldn't sleep for trying to mentally prepare myself for the layoff, even though there is really no way to prepare. It was like getting ready to walk off the plank and fall from the tallest towers of the Emerald City into a nest of the meanest Witches, with their hard laughs cackling in my ears.

In the morning, I put my levis on, added my cowgirl belt, slid into my western shirt and pulled on my boots. Then I walked into the Witch's den. It didn't matter that I had seven years of good standing at the Big hospital. All they cared about was the last six months at their hospital.

I walked up the stairs into a big auditorium-type

The Yellow "Sick" Road

room where all the big chiefs, HR, DON, and management personnel sat with their Witch's smiles. I don't remember what they said. I just took their little termination of employment paper and walked out. I wanted to yell, "Hypocrites!" but I didn't say a word.

I drove away, beside myself, not knowing who to call or if I should just start yelling and crying. If there had been a cliff nearby, I may have driven off it. Nothing made sense in my tumultuous state of mind.

Then I thought of a friend I could call, a friend as tough as the root that helped pull me out of the ditch. Even though she had a lot of health problems, she was spiritually strong and had a lot of faith in God. When I called her, I was crying so hard I couldn't talk.

She kept repeating, "God loves you, and somehow things will work out ok." She also said a prayer for me while we were on the phone. I really believe that she was my guardian angel at that time. I will forever be appreciative that she was there for me when I needed her.

I was 62 years old. Deep down I knew I was a good person and a good nurse and that God loved me. I still needed to work, but couldn't think of

The Ditch

anybody who was going to hire a nurse who should be retiring. But retiring to what? There was no place like home, but how was I going to keep my old pioneer home refuge?

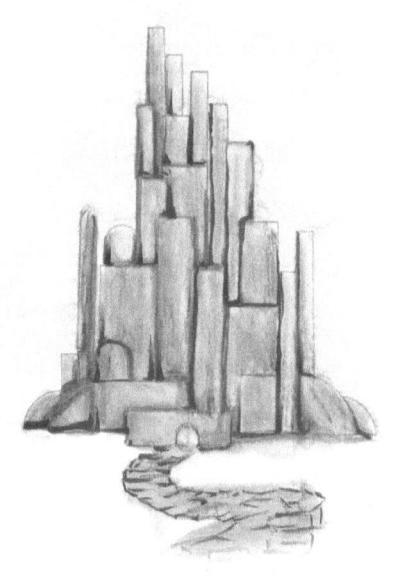

Chapter Ten: Washington DC

Said one of the nurses,
"I'd rather be a Ho!"

I received some severance pay, which was not enough to get me through retirement, but it was enough to keep me afloat until I could figure out what to do. I went to my place of worship and prayed a lot.

I had kept the documentation that my counselor

suggested, but in order to receive my severance pay, I had to sign an agreement that I would not retaliate in any way for being laid off. This meant I could not use any of my notes regarding the abuse I observed.

One thing I believe is that miracles happen. When I felt like I was in the ditch—and I turned things over to God, saying, "Ok, God, I've done everything I can do so now I need a miracle"—that's when miracles happened.

A week after the layoff, I walked into my kitchen and heard the phone ring. (This phone-ringing thing could make a person paranoid.) I picked it up and heard a recording saying, "Please call immediately if you are interested in working a strike in Washington D.C."

I said to myself, *This could be great. It would really help me, because working nursing strikes pays good money.* I'd never worked a strike before and it sounded a little scary, but it could be fun to go to Washington D.C. Besides, I felt I had no choice, so I was game to seize the opportunity if the company would hire me.

The next thing I knew, I was looking out the window of an airplane as we flew over patriotic

The Yellow "Sick" Road

landmarks, such as the White House and the Washington Monument.

Once I landed safely, a van picked me and the other strike nurses up from the airport and took us to a really nice Homestead Suite. It was beautiful, and everybody treated us like VIP'S.

Every day we were bussed through the ghetto up to the Biggest hospital 1 had ever seen- a 700-bed facility in the middle of downtown Washington D.C. Again the thought came that this could be the Emerald City hospital and I would meet the wonderful Oz who would know all the answers to how to be a good nurse without being abused.

The travel nurses gathered in the bus with an air of anticipation and excitement. There were nurses of every nationality and color. I could hardly understand some of them who spoke with southern accents. It didn't matter that there were fat, skinny, beautiful, and homely nurses because we were united for the same cause. When I mentioned that this was my first strike, a couple of nurses took me under their wings.

We had to walk across a picket line, which put us on the television news. That first day, all 200 of us marched like soldiers into a big auditorium. After I sat

Washington DC

down, a nurse announced through a microphone that we were going to have a math test the next day. She said everybody had to get 100%. If they didn't, they would be flown home.

Math has never been my strong subject, and I hadn't studied it much since my nursing boards exam 15 years earlier. The nurse continued, "Here is a study guide for all of you to study tonight. Remember, you must get 100%."

I didn't get much sleep that night as I frantically went over the study guide, trying to figure it out. I studied with an intelligent nurse who knew all the answers, and was grateful for her help. After she went to sleep, my sleep-deprived brain pictures visions of flying back home in humiliation, which didn't help me sleep much.

Walking into the auditorium the next day reminded me of when I took my Boards and had to pass the two-day test in order to be a nurse. I followed my study partner inside, hoping her knowledge would rub off on me. After all the nurses were instructed to sit as far apart from one another as the room allowed, the tests were passed out. We were permitted to use a calculator, but it was their calculator, which made it

The Yellow "Sick" Road

feel a little different, and anything a little different added to my stress. We had to show our written work, and the test was timed, which added pressure, too. I wondering if this was how homeless people felt when they stole to feed their children.

After enduring to the end, I handed in my test and waited anxiously for the results. I was thrilled to learn I had passed the test.

On the way back to our apartments, I took a deep breath as the bus rolled through the ghettos. The cherry blossoms on the trees looked so beautiful that I finally relaxed. There is something about nature that helps put us humans at ease. My perspective on life changed to viewing our planet as a world of wonder. None of us nurses talked—most just fell asleep and let the bus driver do the work.

My first day at the huge hospital was quite amazing. *Emerald City, here I come.* We got off the bus and went into the hospital, walking down a long hall to the nurse's staffing office. Since this was actually a prestrike situation, which means that we were there to take over if the strike didn't settle, the regular nurses didn't want us there and probably had thoughts of sabotage. We all knew it was going to be a brutal contract as we listened to the head nurse give us our assignments for the day.

I rode the elevator to the 7th floor, took a deep breath, and said a silent prayer. I had a gut feeling this wasn't going to be like the Emerald City waiting for me Over the Rainbow.

I asked a group of nurses where I could put my belongings. One pointed vaguely and said, "Over there." The nurse I'd been assigned to train with was so busy that I ended up merely following her around, trying to see where everything was and learn what I was supposed to do. Tomorrow, I'd be on my own. I sensed that this might be a dangerous situation not only for me, but for the patients.

This assignment made me feel like I was on the Civil War battlefield, especially after I was moved to the trauma unit, where I handled patients with gunshot wounds as well as every disease I could imagine. At one point, I walked into a room to see a large patient standing on his bed, not only with IV lines hanging down from his limbs, but the dressing from his abdominal gunshot wound missing.

The Yellow "Sick" Road

Apparently confused, he looked like an accident waiting to happen. Since he was too big for me to handle alone, I called a Code Gray, pushing a bedside phone button to alert an emergency team.

In ten minutes, several large men entered the room and restrained him with leather straps, securing him to his bed. I called the doctor, who ordered me to sedate him. Once he was calm, I redressed his wound.

One unusual experience for me is that I was usually the only Caucasian in sight. There were times when the charge nurse would see me at the end of the hall and call out, "Sanborn, get down here!" By the time I hurried to her station, she claimed to have forgotten why she called me. I wonder if she just wanted to see me hurry at her command.

That night, we travel nurses got on the bus to return to our hotel. One big nurse suddenly pushed herself wearily to her feet and shouted, "I'd rather be a ho (whore)!"

We all knew the strike would not be easy money when we took the assignment. During my eight-week contract, I had some of the best and some of the worst medical experiences of my career.

When my contract was up, my cowboy husband,

Washington DC

Scott, came to Washington to pick me up. He's the one who taught me to love horses and camping, and he also appreciated my pioneer home, which made him a keeper. We had a fun vacation together, traveling to New York, visiting Times Square, monuments, museums, and historical battlefields.

My career has changed the way I think of the medical world. While this hospital wasn't like the Emerald City I envisioned, in a way, it served the purpose of the Emerald City. I realized that I was becoming my own Oz by learning things for myself. As I traveled the Yellow Sick Road, I was obtaining answers through my own experience on how to become the best nurse I could be.

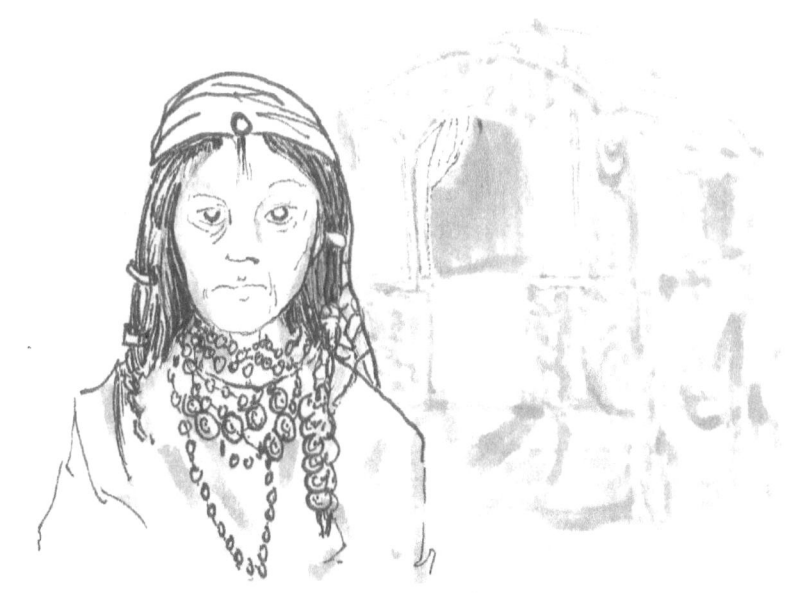

Chapter Eleven: The Gypsy

"At least I knew if I woke up,
I wasn't dead."

My character-building experience during the Washington D.C. strike helped me get a lot of confidence back. In spite of worrying about the test, I hadn't been one of the eight nurses dismissed for not reaching 100%. I had also done a good job of handling situations I'd never encountered before.

Still, there is no place like home. Once I left the east coast, I returned to my home, sweet home to regroup. I had made some good money, so I wasn't so panicky about just grabbing anything I could.

Next I found a northern California travel assignment 11 hours away from my pioneer home. I managed to work this assignment for nearly a year, with my biggest challenge being homesickness. A couple of my sons lived just a few hours away in southern California, so I stayed with one son one weekend, and the other one the next weekend.

When the homesickness grew unbearable, I would drive for 11 hours just to be home for a while. Sometimes I would stop at Mesquite and go to a slot machine, which would sometimes be lucky. I would gamble my entire allotted $10.00. If I won enough for a motel, I would allow myself the comforts of a nice room. If I lost, I would just drive straight through. If I were too exhausted, sometimes I would sleep for a while in the parking lot in my car until I was rested enough to continue on.

The Yellow "Sick" Road

I began feeling a bit sorry for myself while living like a gypsy. I was so displaced that some mornings I had to orientate myself when I woke up. I felt like an "It," a nameless person in another forgettable diner. I longed for routine and familiar surroundings.

Oddly enough, in other ways, traveling made me feel carefree. Yet more often, I felt emotionally exhausted and lonely. In the "Wizard of Oz," Dorothy meets the traveling salesman in his gypsy wagon before becoming the ultimate traveler with her house swept up into the tornado, which sent her to a far-off place where she was surrounded by little people.

Homesickness is like a hollow log - dark and long and empty. If I talked alone in my room, it was like an echo with nobody to listen. When I walked around the motel, nobody knew me nor cared if I was there or not, except the managers who took my rent. I would have taken my two mini poodles, but when I worked the night shift, they wouldn't let me sleep during the day because they'd bark at every little noise. I was afraid their barking would get me kicked out of the motel.

When I was in my motel room, I'd remember

The Gypsy

riding my horse on a little mountain west of my house. Riding was such a comfort. I'd recall sitting in the saddle and feeling the warmth of my horse, her muscles moving beneath me as she carried the gypsy Claudia across the landscape. I loved the smell of my horse and saddle, so in the motel, all I had to do was pretend I could smell them to feel better. If you have ever had a horse, you know what I mean. I loved my horse, and drew deep comfort from thinking of her.

One morning, exhausted from working the night shift, I was stunned when the desk clerk told me I needed to move out of my room because someone else had reserved it. Since my schedule was so crazy and somewhat unpredictable, I just rented a room for a night at a time. The clerk assured me that there was a vacant room available on the third floor.

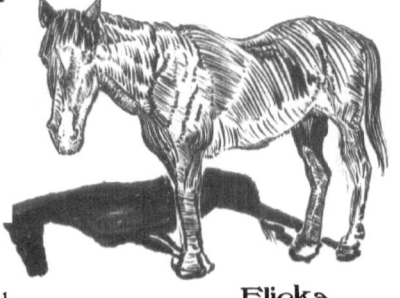

Flicka

After I got my wits about me, I had to lift all my stuff up to the third floor, including my bike. Men who passed by me didn't even offer to help.

When I was finally settled in my room, telling myself I had to hurry and go to sleep so I could get up to work the coming night shift, I had to ask myself - was this job really worth it? I couldn't answer that right away. I needed rest so I could be a good nurse that night.

During this work assignment, I was scheduled to work on Thanksgiving evening, which turned out to be one of the saddest I've ever had.

I was staying with my son in Dana Point, and his wife was cooking their Thanksgiving dinner to be done at 5:00 pm. I'd let them know ahead of time that if they scheduled the dinner at 2:00 pm, then I could share it with them, but she said it couldn't be done. Her tradition was to have Thanksgiving dinner at 5 pm, and she was going to have it at that time with my son and her children (my son's stepchildren.) Nothing was going to interfere with her schedule.

Luckily, I had paid the fare for one of my other sons to travel in order to be with me on Thanksgiving. Together, we went into a homeless shelter church chapel. As I looked around at the poor souls gathered there, I experienced one of the most humbling feelings I'd ever had. I was spending a day that I had always been taught was traditionally for family with strangers who probably had no family to speak of.

The Gypsy

I was reminded of the Beatitude: "Blessed are the poor in spirit, for theirs is the kingdom of heaven." Matt 5:3. I truly feel there is a special place for people who are poor as to the wealth of the world. I'm not going to judge them. I'm sure they all have a story. I remembered what it was like trying to raise my four sons as a single mother, and the times we had no money. We could have easily been homeless ourselves.

There are times now when my husband Scott and I spend Thanksgiving alone, with just the two of us and nowhere else to go, but that's nothing compared to the time my son and I visited the homeless shelter.

One Christmas Eve when my sons were still at home, I worked the night shift while they stayed with their dad. A certain quietness filled the air on the floor I was working, and I ached that I wasn't sharing Christmas Eve with my sons.

I went into the room of one of my patients, a man in his 60's, and he began talking to me. He was a professional man, and explained that he had two sons with such severe mental illness that they had to be institutionalized. As he talked, it appeared to be painful for him to verbalize some of his family issues.

The Yellow "Sick" Road

As I listened to him and his sadness, his words brought comfort to me, as much as I hoped I'd brought to him. His story helped me forget my own pain of working Christmas Eve without my family. I remembered, like an old time video being played, all the past Christmas Eve's spent with my sons and their dad.

Little did I know in the next few years that my own son would have a terrible accident and suffer a life-changing brain injury, and my youngest son would develop mental illness.

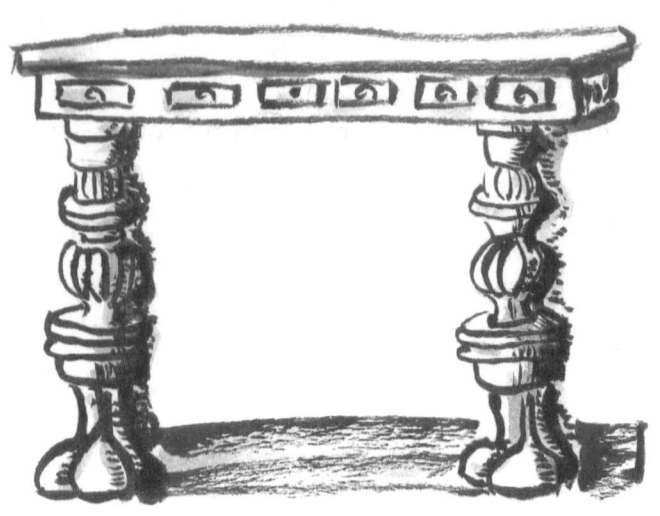

Chapter Twelve: The Desk

A Director of Nursing
not even having a desk?

I had just finished a travel contract and was outside feeding my horse, feeling relief because there's no place like home. I wondered what I would do next to keep myself afloat financially so I could prepare for retirement.

Suddenly, a white car drove onto my horse

The Yellow "Sick" Road

property. I didn't recognize it. A brief thought that it might be a policeman flitted through my mind, and I wondered if I was in trouble.

A young woman who was a stranger to me got out of the car and walked toward me. As she explained that someone who knew someone who knew me had suggested that she might find me by my horse, I wondered if maybe she was interested in buying a horse. Finally, she got to the point.

She had come on behalf of a care center in a nearby town, and invited me to come and interview for a job as a Director of Nurses.

I was stunned. I had never heard of this rehab care center. How often does anyone, let alone a nurse, have someone come and look for them on an acre of land kept for horses to extend an invitation for a job? Feeling a bit distrustful, I took her name and phone number and said I would look into it. If I were interested, I'd call and schedule an interview.

Still, I couldn't help feeling a little flattered that she was seeking me out to be a director.

Being the religious person I am, I can be a little mystical at times. I thought for one moment that perhaps the young lady was the Witch of the East in

The Desk

disguise, and had come to drag me to the Emerald City along the Yellow Sick Road.

At last I decided to take a chance. I had been a director two other times, and an assistant director for two years, so I was confident that I was qualified for the job.

Before making the phone call to arrange an interview, I imagined putting my silver-white nurse slippers on and clicking them three times to see if they would carry me to a wonderful place to work. I pictured the ability to go to work close by and return home every night. I fantasized having an office with a desk made of emerald stones, with eager Flying Monkeys coming to my aide. I imagined working with aides I wouldn't have to go looking for in closets. Interactions with the Wizard of Oz (the administrator) would result in all the answers I needed to be brave, courageous, and smart enough to run the Emerald City (the Rehab Care Center) perfectly. The Munchkin patients would be so happy, and their care would be perfect. I would truly believe

The Yellow "Sick" Road

in the knowledge that, "If I ever go looking for my heart's desire again, I won't look any further than my own backyard," because home is a place created within yourself.

I researched the facility and found that it did not have the best ratings. It was one star out of a possible five. That was a red flag, which meant that this place was probably very dysfunctional. Yet I said to myself, "Oh, what the heck. What do I have to lose?"

I picked up the phone and called the facility. After a moment's hesitation, I introduced myself and related how the young woman had invited me to interview for a job as a Director of Nursing. I went ahead and made the interview appointment, hoping that during it a vocera wouldn't go off to say, "Don't hire Claudia Sanborn."

I went out and bought a new suit for the interview. I also studied interview protocol on the Internet.

My review board consisted of seven people. When they introduced themselves, I discovered they were staff members from every ancillary of the care center. They took turns asking me questions. I answered in what I felt was a professionally appropriate manner.

Months later, I found out that after the meeting, they voted as to whether they wanted me or not, even though I was the only person interviewing for the position. I also found out that most of them voted for me because if they didn't, they were afraid they were going to be under the jurisdiction of a new graduate RN whom they hated. Apparently, she had a Wicked Witch of the West reputation, and had declared that she wanted this position and was going to get it no matter what. She'd been working as an LPN (Licensed Practical Nurse) staff nurse, and had just passed her boards to become the big RN (Registered Nurse).

I also found out that the woman who recruited me was in corporate, and had worked with me when I had been an ADON under the DON who was stealing drugs.

I got the job.

The first day of my employment, the new RN and the administrator talked to me for several hours about how terrible all the nurses were. It was a very negative meeting, insinuating that they wanted me to fire all of them. I asked the administrator who was going to take care of the patients if I fired all those nurses. When a facility is short staffed, the ADON and DON work the floor. It makes no sense for management to work the floor because there aren't any nurses.

Little did they know I was a nurse advocate. I was even part of a committee called Creating a Better Work Environment which was dedicated to making a better environment in the nursing workforce and legislate against bullying.

Shaking my head to myself, I thought, *What have I gotten myself into now?*

Since I had no intention of firing the nurses, it was no surprise to discover that I was very popular with the nurses and aides. They all loved me and thought I was their savior. I was like the kind Witch of the South rescuing them from the mean Witch of the West. It was not uncommon for them to pull me aside and tell me how happy they were that I was there. I thought that if I had a team behind me, it had to work. *How could I go wrong?*

But I also discovered that the newly graduated

The Desk

RN was best friends with the administrator. After a few months, it began to seem as if they had only hired me to appease corporate. It was beginning to feel like a setup. The new RN had her stuff all over the desk I was supposed to use, and she was not about to give it up. Several times I asked the administrator how I could do my job without a desk. She said, "Oh, we are working on it. We are trying to find a place for you."

Wait a minute—I'm second to the top in command of this whole care center and they are not giving me enough respect to be able to use my desk? Think about it: a desk is where work gets organized. It has drawers and compartments to put paper clips, rubber bands, pens, pencils, erasers, computers, telephones, papers, etc. A desk is where successful organization takes place with files and documents. A desk is where people know to go to make contact and communicate. Yet here I was, working on a corner of the desk that had been taken over by someone who wanted my job!

I was tired of being put off with excuses like,

The Yellow "Sick" Road

"Oh, maybe by Monday." After several weeks of orientation and no desk, I didn't know how to function efficiently. I even called HR and corporate to let them know what was going on.

I determined to continue going to the administrator to try and develop camaraderie. Every morning I went in and visited with her, sometimes indirectly hinting about the desk. When I talked to her about the problems, she said there was nothing she could do. Things just got worse when the new RN felt threatened by my attention to her friend.

Still, I really wanted this job to work.

There was a big important corporate meeting at the Little American Hotel in Salt Lake City. It was festive, and all the management and directors were treated like royalty and given the red carpet treatment. This type of welcome was really starting to make me feel more secure. My old administrator from the facility where the DON did drugs was there, and he bragged about me and said I was very competent.

The administrator escorted me to the hospital next door to the care center so I could meet all the doctors. This was an encouraging experience, and I felt like I was making progress.

The Desk

One morning I bravely walked into the administrator's office and said that if I didn't have a desk by Monday, I might as well not come in. She said I could move everything that belonged to the RN off her desk and put it on a different desk that would be brought in.

That went over like a bomb. Now the new grad nurse was so angry she wouldn't speak to me. I just ignored her and did my job, even though my workplace was getting kind of uncomfortable.

The RN worked harder to sabotage me, and I worked harder to get in good with the administrator and staff. But ultimately, the good ole boy thing prevailed. The RN and administrator had known each other for years and lived in the same town.

Five months into my employment, the administrator began leaving me out of meetings and not consulting me on decision-making. It was more traumatizing than I thought it would be. When staff pulled me aside to whisper, "Watch your back," I began having nightmares.

One day, a male corporate nurse

came out to monitor the facility. The new RN was so suggestive and flirtatious, inviting him to go to her house if he needed anything, that it was embarrassing. They were often together alone, and I'm sure he got an earful of how awful I was, and that all the nurses needed to be fired.

I didn't have a chance. He sided with her, even though when he gave me a list of assignments, I did them all and turned them in on time. When he gave the RN a list, she only did about half of her assignments, probably because she was too busy flirting.

When a resident patient blamed an aide for multiple problems, a vote was taken as to whether to keep or fire the aide. I voted to keep her, but I lost the vote and the aide was fired.

I called corporate and informed them of how I felt about the situation. The next thing I knew, I was called in to the administrator's office to a conference call.

I wasn't worried, but I should have been.

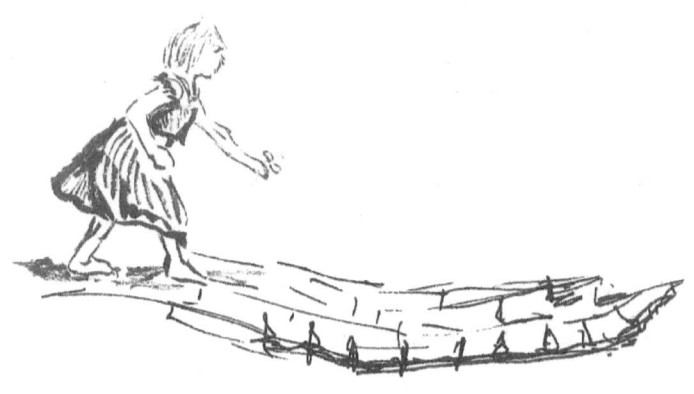

Chapter Thirteen: Pending Doom

Repeatedly Sweeping the Yellow Sick Road

Does anyone know how to explain the feeling of pending doom, of facing walking the plank again? I know there are a lot of readers out there who understand what rejection feels like, because it comes in too many ways to mention.

I gave it my best effort and tried to stay. I really wanted to retain those nurses and save corporate a lot

The Yellow "Sick" Road

of money. Research shows that constantly hiring and firing costs thousands of dollars.

I tried with all my heart, courage, and brain to succeed in all of my jobs. The only thing that saves me is knowing that I have been true to myself. I defended this aide, speaking up when I felt the resident was suffering from emotional problems and depression that led to accusing the aide falsely. Then I lost my job. Management had been overheard swearing about the aide in the hall, and yet the aide was brought in and confronted about her swearing in front of the resident. It was a double standard—"Do as I say, but not as I do." Even to this day, I believe that this aide does not know I defended her, and that defense was the straw that broke the camel's back.

One thing that helps to handle the confusion in my life is that I live in a beautiful, calming area. While driving to work on that fateful day, I watched lambs grazing on green hills and noticed the sun coming up to spread its rays over the still, quiet morning.

As I pulled into the parking lot and rolled into the space I always parked in, I pondered my agenda for the day. What should I start on first? There is some comfort in routine.

I walked down the hall and into my office and sat down at my desk. I took a deep breath before delving into my day's agenda.

Then my phone rang. It was the administrator calling me into her office. The thought of termination entered my mind, but I felt like they would surely write me a warning first. I hadn't been counseled at all, but there had been many disagreements with the administrator and the nurse who wanted my job. Still, I felt a bit of security that I was the second in command. Having held this job for six months gave me a little bit of reassurance, too. I had a desk now. That had to mean something.

When I walked into the administrator's office, it felt different than before. It was uncomfortable. In spite of this, I said, "Hi." She smiled and asked me to close the door and sit down. Then she told me that corporate was on the phone as a tele-conference.

I thought that was ok because we were probably having a threesome meeting. I picked up the phone and discovered that the HR representative on

The Yellow "Sick" Road

the line was the same one I had talked to about the aide being falsely accused of mistreating the resident. I had thought he was my friend and confidante until he told me that I was going to be terminated. He said I'd falsely accused the administrator of firing the aide and saying she'd been used as a scapegoat.

I just listened. In the back of my mind I realized I'd been wondering how they were going to do this, and now I knew. They had finally found something to use to let me go. The new RN had finally managed to get me out of there. I had been set up and they had won.

I said, "OK," and walked out, down the long hallway back to my office, and looked at my desk that I had so diligently fought for. What a waste. Chalk this up to another learning experience along the Yellow Sick Road. I really believe I was doomed to fail before I even started the job, because the administrator was just trying to appease corporate by hiring me, when she really wanted the new RN to have the job.

Embarrassed and humiliated, I packed my things from the desk, then walked quietly out to my car. My heart was hurting badly. I really wanted to hug all the nurses and residents who loved me. I had again gotten attached to all these people, but now I just had to get out of there.

Management just doesn't have a clue how unjust termination ruins people.

As I drove home, I recalled a discussion in my Creating a Better Work Environment committee about a person who killed himself after being terminated. This guy had a family, and being fired was too much for him to face.

This experience taught me not to take just any job. A big red flag was having to fight for a simple desk. That's when I should have seen what was coming. I felt like the scapegoat for the administrator and the new RN.

I decided to do what I could to lobby for laws requiring training for management personnel. Management should not be allowed to use people. It should be against the law to intentionally harm an employee for the benefit and gain of another employee simply because they are a friend.

I found solace with my horse. I gave her a big hug and started crying as I took in the familiar scent of her fur. Knowing something was wrong, she just stood still and let me hug and pat her. My horse does not gossip and backbite. My mind played over all the beautiful places we had been together, and I suddenly knew there could be a good life after termination. "Thank You, Flicka."

After receiving comfort from my horse, I got back into my car and drove home. Opening the door and walking into my warm, cozy house gave me the feeling of a big hug and the sense that things were ok, because there's no place like home.

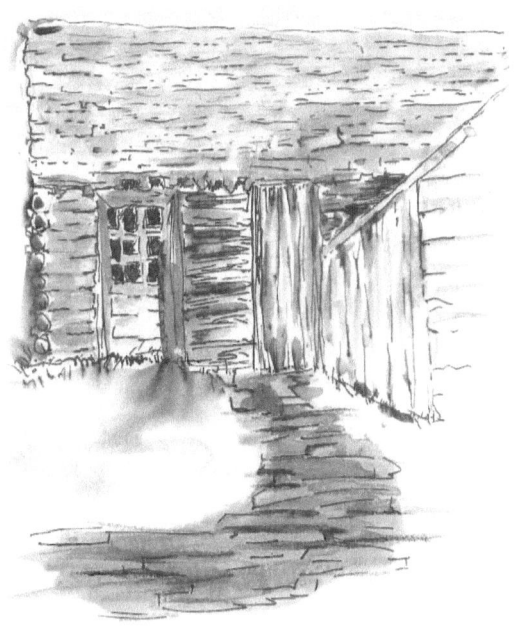

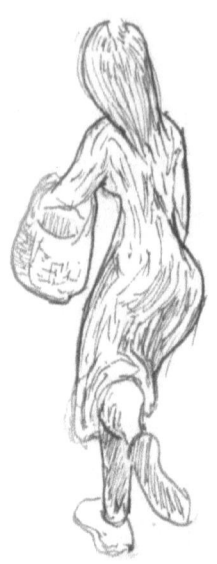

Chapter Fourteen: Religious Emerald City

" Blessed are they that mourn,
for they shall be comforted."
Matthew 5:3-10

Nursing my recent abrasions, scrapes, and bruises, I limped along the Yellow Sick Road toward my next travel assignment at a religious hospital in the High Desert of California. This turned out to be one of the most pleasant places

The Yellow "Sick" Road

to work in regard to teamwork and consideration toward staff. Here, at last, was an Emerald City where the Wizard of Oz was actually polite.

Each shift began with a word of prayer broadcast over the intercom speaker. During shift changes throughout my career, I would sometimes feel nervous perspiration on my forehead while giving my report to the oncoming nurse, because she'd usually be on the lookout to see if the departing nurse was dumping any of unfinished work on her. Most hospital facilities would require both nurses to go to the patients' bedside to make sure they were stable and not declining. The patient IV's would also be checked. It was actually a good idea to follow through with this kind of report for assurance that you were not "dumping," and I was caught off guard when the nurses at the religious hospital didn't find fault with each other at shift changes.

This hospital was not of my religion, but I felt a calm sense of spirituality there. At this point in my career, this atmosphere was a welcome relief and offered me hope that there wouldn't be gossip. The work on the floor was heavy and quite busy, but the charge nurse was willing to answer questions to the best of her ability, without any attitude that she was too busy so everyone else had to figure things out for themselves. The staff also seemed to genuinely appreciate me being there. It was a little like I had imagined it would be when I graduated from nursing school. In fact, if I could have gotten a permanent job there, I might have done it. Word had it that if you were a super nurse, you could possibly be hired.

My life as a nurse at this particular hospital was in control, sort of like a cattle drive, which is hard yet rewarding work. The halls weren't too long or hollow sounding, which could make someone to want to yell, "Hey, is there anyone out there?" I even liked the religious statues everywhere, including the courtyards outside. The images created a warm, compassionate feeling surrounding me.

"Blessed are those that mourn, for they shall be comforted." Matt 5:4. I felt comforted. I didn't have to sweep The Yellow Sick Road this time. I hummed "Somewhere Over the Rainbow" to myself as I walked down the hall. I said a prayer at night in my motel and thanked my God that I had peace and comfort for this time.

The Yellow "Sick" Road

I could actually smell the orange poppies in the air, which gave me a chance to take a deep breath before the next contract. The cute Munchkin patients had moderate diagnoses that did not require calling a doctor or transferring any of them to a more acute floor.

Even though the pay was fair, and there were no ditches or Wicked Witches or Flying Monkeys hiding from their work, I still looked forward to the end of the eight-week contract.

The problem was after I left the Emerald City hospital. I was staying at a reasonably priced motel that felt desolate even though the noisy freeway nearly ran down the middle of it because there was nobody for me to talk to. The town had nothing to offer in the way of entertainment. I know, because I drove around trying to find something to do and there wasn't even a movie theater. One night, the police came because the motel had been robbed, but it didn't even faze me. I had developed a non-feeling sense of just making it through another day.

Religious Emerald City

I was lonely after work was done, but since I was an eight-hour drive from my house, I drove home after work every week, which helped me keep my sanity.

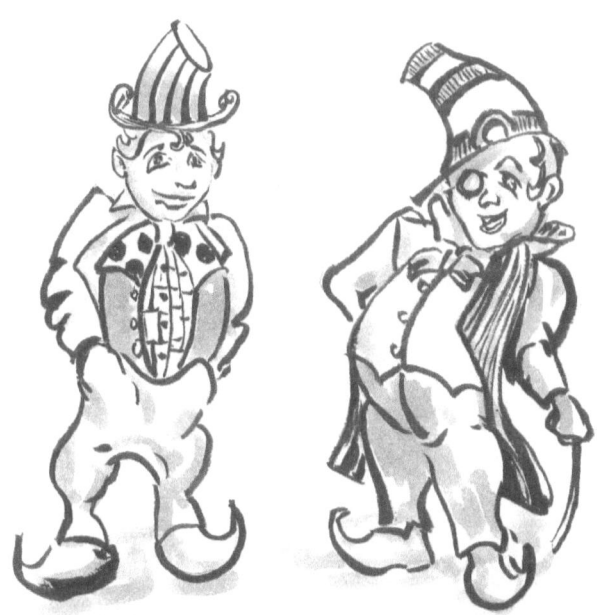

Chapter Fifteen: The Munchkins

Never be so angry in the end
that there's nobody there to
hold your hand during your last breath.

My effort to describe care given to dying patients is intended to generate empathy rather than judgment. Sometimes it's hard to tell how it might seem to others, since I had to create different spaces in my heart to neutralize the pain, yet still allow my heart to continue beating with sufficient rhythm to feel some of the pain my patients felt. This was particularly true when I took care of the sickest of all the sick—cancer patients.

For this challenging assignment, I again packed my necessities and was off to California to a top-notch hospital that housed celebrities and very wealthy patients. By the nature of those who occupied the beds, I anticipated that there would also be good quality hospital staff.

In my customary way of checking things out so the first day would be less overwhelming, the first thing I did on arrival was drive around the hospital, parking facilities, and motels. My gypsy mode kicked in and I settled into the cheapest motel I could find.

The first day of orientation was basically like all the others - get my password, learn the computer, learn how to get into the pyxis for medications, learn how to answer the call light and wear the vocera around my neck, learn how to page other nurses and staff, learn where everything is and the combinations on the doors to get in.

The elevator and halls were not emerald green and I didn't see the aide flying around like a Winged

Monkey. I did not see any Witches, but there was the expected hierarchy of charge nurse and manager.

One thing I loved was that each morning while taking a report, I could look out the window and see the ocean. Just looking at the vast blue stretch of never-ending water helped me keep in perspective that each hour and each day was so important to these patients.

Getting to know my patients was like Dorothy getting acquainted with the Munchkins. In spite of their surroundings, these patients were generally cheerful. They appreciated every new day of life, as well as the new nurse, even though I had appeared as unexpectedly as Dorothy dropping in on Oz. As I helped them make each day the best it could be, I realized that this was one time in my twenty-two years of nursing that I felt like I really made a difference.

Sometimes when I walked into patients' rooms, their faces glowed with happiness at the sight of me. In spite of the disease taking over their bodies, they still had a special feeling of hope. As I turned and adjusted them for comfort, I tried the best I could not to add to their pain. I would use pillows to help take pressure off their brittle bones and flaccid muscles.

The Munchkins

They appreciated everything I did and treated me like I was an angel from heaven. Their loved ones and family members in the room also never gave up the hope that their loved ones would get well. All they wanted was one more day, one more hour.

Yet there was one patient with a different view, which made her unforgettable. The tall, attractive African American lady was on her last few days of hospice care (care for easing symptoms of the terminally ill.) She did not want any visitors: no family, no friends. Angry with everybody and everything, she stayed alone in her room. Visible from the nurse's station, we looked in on her lying on her back in the dark, empty room. She refused to let us turn her or do anything else that might ease her suffering. She insisted that she wanted to die alone, her wrinkled brow plainly showing her attitude toward life. Her spirit had died in that lifeless room before her body had even stopped working. I wanted to shake her to give her some emotion. I wanted her to have hope like so many of my other patients had, yet she remained angry and silent. It was the saddest experience I had ever witnessed.

Years earlier, I'd made a commitment that if I

The Yellow "Sick" Road

had a dying patient, I would not let them die alone, because I don't want to go that way. I want someone to be there to hold my hand. I don't really care who it is---just don't want to leave this world without someone at my side.

Because of my strong feelings for Memorial Day, one of my sons has made a commitment to put flowers on my grave at least that single day of the year. I think it's important that a family member or friend cares enough to commemorate a loved one's life just one day of the year.

I didn't get a chance to hold the lonely cancer patient's hand. One day when I returned to work, I learned that she had died in the night. When I saw her empty room, which was no less empty than when she was in it, a lump rose in my throat. As I glanced at the other nurses, I sensed their sadness. Oncology nurses have a compassionate disposition, which makes it hard for them not to get attached to their patients.

On the opposite end of the spectrum, one of the more hopeful patients wore a different wig every time I went into her room. Her make up was always carefully applied to the wrinkled skin stretched over her sunken cheeks. The nightgowns and robes she

The Munchkins

wore from home were always fresh, clean, and beautiful. She insisted that she put on fresh, clean clothing every day, and always looked the best she could. She was elderly —but she had a boyfriend. What a compliment to her! Even though she was a big time fall risk, she was bound and determined to do everything herself. She was alert and always wanted to talk, as though it was her mission to cheer up the nurses so they would have a good day.

It was a joy to take care of such a special Munchkin. Her courage and attitude was such a great example to me. I pictured her when she died as an angel floating around the clouds and waving to us down here. Her spirit was so strong that she would probably stay around to help boost the spirits of the other dying patients on the floor.

There is a disadvantage to being a travel nurse, because even though you try not to get attached to those you work with, it still happens. When this cancer ward contract was over, I was truly sad. I missed the staff and patients more than the view of the ocean. The only benefit from being a temporary employee was that I didn't have to deal with the politics.

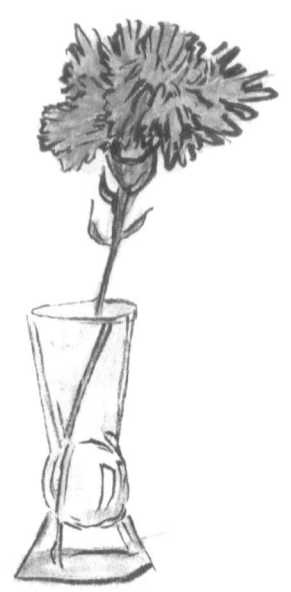

Chapter Sixteen: Vase with a Red Carnation

It wasn't orange poppies—
but it was the next best thing

One of my favorite travel assignments took place in California in a small, rural hospital located in a poor part of California. Sometimes small hospitals are the hardest to work

The Yellow "Sick" Road

because if you are the only one available, you have to wear a lot of hats and cover what needs to be done, whether you're qualified or not.

I couldn't see the beach from the hospital window, but when my shift ended, I could take a ten-minute drive to arrive at a beautiful, calm, blue beach. It was different from the sunny, populated beaches I was most familiar with. This was a wonderfully remote, quiet, misty beach where I could relax after working several 12-hour shifts. A long old rickety pier stretched out into the waves, which sometimes washed up so high that it gave me the feeling that if I stood on it, it could break into a million pieces and I'd be washed ashore.

Being in a poor area worked to my advantage because it also offered low-cost motel rates. There were also a lot of homeless people on the streets and murals painted on cinderblock buildings. Rather than graffiti, the artwork appeared to be done by good artists and showed historical images of the town, including patriotic scenes and flowerpots in windows. These pictures made me feel an attachment to the community, even though I knew my working assignment would be over soon and I didn't want to get too fond of a place I'd be leaving.

During my nine-month hospital contract, I met a nurse around my age who was rumored to be divorced from a doctor who'd run off with a younger nurse. This woman was fairly attractive for her age, with a petite frame and thick, graying blonde hair. She could have dated if she wanted to, but she said she didn't need a man. Instead, she lost herself in the care and welfare of her patients. Work was her whole world. She would come in any time they called her, competent to float to all the different units in the hospital.

She was very helpful with any questions I had about learning the new computer system and where everything was. She even invited me to her home. I was impressed by her small mansion until I realized that it felt empty and hollow inside. It didn't seem as if she'd moved anything that was there since her husband left. She never talked about her ex-husband and appeared to be over the trauma, but speaking from experience, I don't think anyone ever really gets over a divorce.

During my first week of work, I couldn't help but notice little red carnations placed around the

The Yellow "Sick" Road

hospital in little glass medicine bottles that had been painted with fun little scenes. They were so cute that I started asking who had made these little vases and filled them with flowers. I wasn't surprised to discover that it was the single nurse who'd made work her life. She'd gather the bottles after the medication had been distributed and take them home to paint. Then she brought them back for volunteers to fill with carnations.

These cheerful little vases set a cheerful tone to the whole floor, which seemed to help in creating an atmosphere that made people treat each other with extra consideration. Not once did I notice any backbiting. In fact, the charge nurse told me that people who gossiped could be written up for it. Yes! Finally, this little hospital had caught on to the real spirit of nursing.

There was no Wicked Witch anywhere in sight. The charge nurse made every attempt to make fair assignments, along with an explanation of why she matched patients with nurses. The aides appeared before you even thought you needed them, like Flying Monkeys to the rescue. My assignment was repeatedly extended, and the charge nurse told me often that she was pleased with my work. I believe they may have offered me a permanent job, but they were looking for someone with more longevity. They appeared to anticipate that I would be retiring soon. Little did they know how much this job meant to me.

My heart ached when it was finally time to pack up my stuff and leave for the last time. I had tears in my eyes when I said good-bye and left with good references from both the charge nurse and the wonderful nurse who created the little vases for the red carnations. But most important of all, I regained my faith in nurses and management. There was a little of the Emerald City at this hospital, which offered me the courage, heart, and brains necessary to carry on.

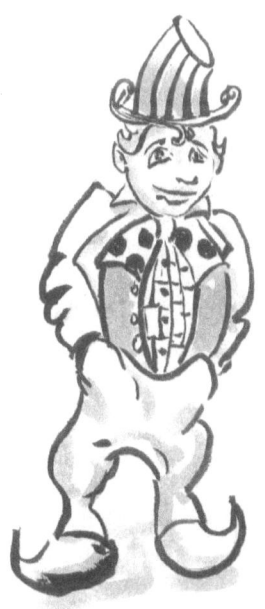

Chapter Seventeen: The Confession

"Please help me!"

Although not a bullying incident, the experience I had with a dying patient is worth mentioning to illustrate what goes on with patient care from a nurse's point of view. We as nurses never know what our patients' needs will be from hour to hour. One minute we could have a life-

The Confession

threatening emergency, and the next thing a patient is emotionally distraught about his life and is afraid to die. Whatever the need, I wanted to be there.

This particular day I clocked in as usual. When I got the outgoing nurse's report, she explained that a certain patient kept obsessing over and over that he was going to die. He was on the rehabilitation unit, and although he had a little history of a heart condition, he was not symptomatic and had no chest pain, yet he was sure he was going to die right away. He wouldn't stop saying that he was going to die that night. His wife was very attentive and came in to see him daily, but she wasn't there.

We are always told to listen to our patients because they know themselves better than anyone else. This 60-year-old patient asked every nurse who went into his room to sit down and listen to him confess about what he had done throughout his life.

When I finished hearing the report, I looked up the patient's medical history on his chart. I also checked his labs to see if anything had been overlooked that might make him more fragile than he appeared, but I didn't find anything.

We were a little confused as to how to handle

this. It was a bit awkward because his thoughts were scattered and he wanted to tell every nurse about how he had messed around with another lady while he was in Europe. He was very tearful, insisting that she was so beautiful he just couldn't help it. He insisted that he had to talk about the details, but he was very needy and it was hard to make the time to sit down and listen to him. He really needed a lot of empathy, and appreciated every minute I could spare so he could talk. A lot of the nurses were getting frustrated and exhausted with him. A few of the staff just rolled their eyes when they came out of the room.

I had my own opinion regarding his affair, but it wasn't my job to judge, or my calling as a nurse to forgive. I tried to simply listen and try to be objective and not get emotionally involved. It was hard to be a therapeutic listener for him---but this is what, as a professional, I was taught to do.

I finally asked if he minded if we called the Chaplain, and he said that was just what he needed. I also made arrangements for a social worker to come in and give him counseling. I was relieved to see the Chaplain go into the room. I think seeing the professionals helped him, because after they left, he

The Confession

talked about what the Chaplain and social worker said to him.

As I clocked out that day, I planned to check on this patient as early as I could on my next shift to see if he'd made it through the night.

The next day after I quietly walked down the hall and peeked into the patient's room, I saw that he was still there, breathing. Imagine that! I went in and said, "Hi. I'm glad you made it through the night." He seemed a little embarrassed. It appeared that he'd decided he was not going to die right away. I didn't bring up the process of his confession, but I think it's what he needed to do the night before.

Then his wife came in, so calm and matter-of-factly that I couldn't tell whether or not she knew about his confession, but I don't think it mattered, because the patient seemed a lot more peaceful.

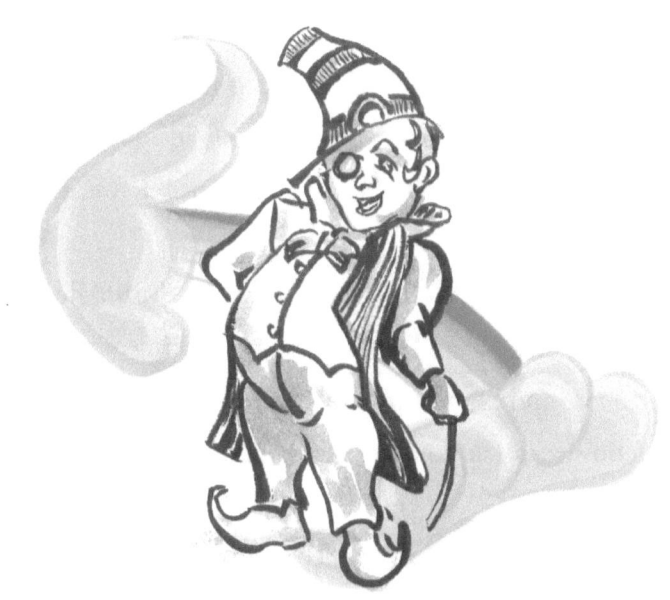

Chapter Eighteen: Dying

When I'm on my last breath, please let me hum softly to myself, "Somewhere Over the Rainbow."

Death represents the ending of something, such as death of relationships or death of loved ones such as mothers and fathers.

I've experienced many types of death, but this chapter will address the first one that I encountered while I was still doing my nurse clinicals.

Dying

Nursing was new to me. No one in my family had anything to do with the medical field, so I wasn't familiar with medical terminology until I went to nursing school.

This particular day, I was working the floor, which means I was learning from working with an instructor and another nurse. I felt like the Scarecrow traveling to an unknown future and learning things along the way.

Then my instructor pulled me aside and told me I was being assigned to a patient in her 80's who was dying. I had mixed feelings, since I'd never seen anyone die before.

When I went into her room to do a morning assessment, my patient was awake and responsive. Her glowing white hair seemed to frame a radiant face, although another part of her seemed to be like a wounded bird. I had an impulse to pat her head and tell her it was going to be okay. Instead, I took her blood pressure and vital signs. Her respiration was slow and irregular, and her heart rate was fast, which meant that the end was near. This was a rare and new experience for me, so I was curious. Would I see her spirit rise to the ceiling, or what?

The Yellow "Sick" Road

I don't know why none of her family members were present. Usually, a patient this close to death is surrounded by loved ones trying to get in one last hug and one last word of goodbye. But this room was quiet, except for the sound of the patient's rapid breathing, which slowed before accelerating again. In spite of this, she was able to answer the questions I was required to ask from my clinical assignment sheet. "What was one of the most memorable experiences you've ever had?"

She replied, "Red Cross" before mumbling something about helping wounded soldiers in the Army. As she spoke, her eyes lit up and her face brightened like an angel. She looked almost translucent as she tried to keep on speaking, but no more words would come. Her expression said it all. Then I sat in a chair beside her bed and held her hand so she wouldn't be alone when she died.

Experiences like this can uproot past memories, making me wonder if perhaps the reason I didn't want anyone to be lonely came from my experience as a frightened little girl waiting for my parents to stop one of their nights of having a party. They drank some at parties, and when I was little, I didn't

Dying

understand peoples' strange behavior when they drank that weird smelling alcohol. Sometimes from my young point of view, I was afraid that my parents might desert me, leaving me all alone to fend for myself. When I was afraid, I would crawl into bed with my big sister and lie there, unable to quit shaking.

My mother was a sixteen-year-old bride, and my father was stationed in Germany for two years during World War II. After he returned, I was born when my mother was twenty-one, making me a Baby Boomer.

In a lot of respects, my childhood was fun and carefree, but there were plenty of times when I felt scared. There were times as a little girl when I was starving. With my dad going to college on the GI Bill, there just wasn't a lot of extra food lying around. I remember eating a lot of Campbell's soup, but I would climb on the roof so I could reach the plums that grew on an overhanging branch. I also picked rhubarb and chewed on the stalks to ease my hunger.

To deal with my feelings of insecurity, I sucked my thumb for too many years. My parents put awful-tasting stuff on my thumb, but that didn't stop me. Even when I started school, I took every opportunity to take a sneaky suck on my thumb because it was such a comfort.

My haunting feeling of loneliness at various times in my uncertain childhood made it so that I never wanted a person to be lonely, which included seeing anyone dying alone. I just didn't want this patient to be alone in her last hours. So I held her hand and counted her breaths and charted them on my assessment papers.

Unfortunately, this patient did not pass away on my shift. I hope someone held her hand when she died.

When I came back the next day, it was weird to glance into her room and see it vacant. I just sighed and kept on walking, trying to process the sad, scary, and marvelous elements of this new experience along the Yellow Brick Road.

Everyone faces death differently. My close friend remembers her grandmother singing all the church songs she knew at the top of her lungs when she was close to dying. I sometimes imagine myself humming under my breath, "Somewhere Over the Rainbow" before I take my last breath. I hope by then I will have forgotten how I couldn't find some of the Flying

Dying

Monkeys when I needed help, or Oz who had no answers for me. Please, by then let the world know how much bullying and cruelty there is in the workforce, especially in the medical field.

This book is for the public and legislature to make changes. Please, on my way back home while traveling down the Yellow Sick Road, may I learn to forgive. I want my heart to be as loving as the Tin Man's in the Wizard of Oz.

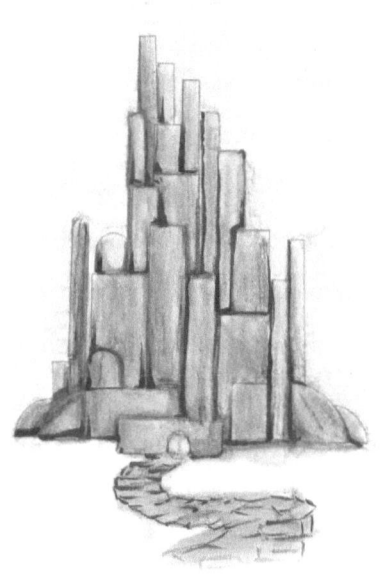

Chapter Nineteen: Really Scary

"UM-HUM"

One night a really scary thing happened to me on the 5th floor at the University Hospital in California, which was located in a rather slummy part of town. When I look back, I think it may have been more dangerous than I first thought.

I was working the night shift as a fairly new nurse. The only staff working on this particular unit with me was an aide I was familiar with and another registry aide that had been pulled in from an agency. In the medical field, you get to know familiar faces even if you don't necessarily know their names, but this registry aide was unfamiliar to me.

He was tall and dark, and every time I sat down to chart my patients in the computer, he would sit too close beside me and make noises that sounded like he was eating his favorite dessert. As he made the noise, "Um-hum," he'd look me over, checking me out from head to toe. If I moved to another computer, he'd sit too close to me again and repeat, "Um-hum." If I got up to check on patients, he followed me into the room. If the patient was asleep, I'd feel trapped. I couldn't depend on a patient to save me from him—after all, I was there to help the patient.

This floor was eerie anyway because of its seclusion from the rest of the hospital, giving it the potential to be a forgotten area. It was old, with flickering lights and creaking floors. The old walls and odd smells made a person feel that it was haunted. It was a scary place to work anyway, and it was made even more so when this male aide began stalking me.

His behavior continued throughout the night. I

The Yellow "Sick" Road

didn't know what to say to him, so I just kept looking at the clock, waiting for my shift to be over, and tried not to let myself get cornered.

I told the other aide that he was scaring me, but she didn't act like it was a big deal. I was on my own. My back-up plan if he made a move was to scream or run to the patient's phone or desk phone and call security.

Then, while I was in the restroom, I heard him try to open the door. His faint "Um-hum" heard through the door made me shiver with revulsion. Thankfully, the door was locked, but I was afraid to come out. When I heard his footsteps move away, I hurried out of the restroom and dashed to the safety of the nurse's station.

Finally, the night was over. I was lucky that I never saw that agency aide again.

Another frightening event that happened in this big University hospital was because of a gang member who'd suffered a paralyzing injury from a bullet in his back. While he had a steady flow of other gang members coming in and going out of his room, I overheard him talking about how he could hardly wait to get out so he could finish the job.

Really Scary

The pattern for these gang members seemed to be one weekend there'd be a patient in the ER who was a Blood, and the next weekend a Crip would end up in the hospital. My fear was that the opposite gang members would come in and have a big shootout within the hospital walls. Listening to the gang member's plans for retaliation made me decided that my back-up plan for gang warfare was to hide under the nurse's desk if the bullets started flying.

I once had responsibility for a patient in shackles. This patient liked doing art to the point that he had a lot of pictures he'd drawn stacked up at his bedside. His body looked like one big painting with tattoos from the top of his head to his toes.

He liked talking about why he was there, sounding almost proud to tell me that he'd been incarcerated for drugs. He belonged to the Hell's Angels motorcycle gang, which was a different organization when this took place in the 1960's than the people who drive Harley Davidson motorcycles these days. Rumor had it that they had sex orgies and were like a cult.

One other patient in shackles screamed at me that he was in imprisoned for rape. The guard who was with him in the room at all times pulled me aside and warned me to be careful when passing his meds to him, and to keep as much distance from him as possible.

Although all of these incidents were very scary to me, I feel like they helped me develop more courage, like Oz's Cowardly Lion.

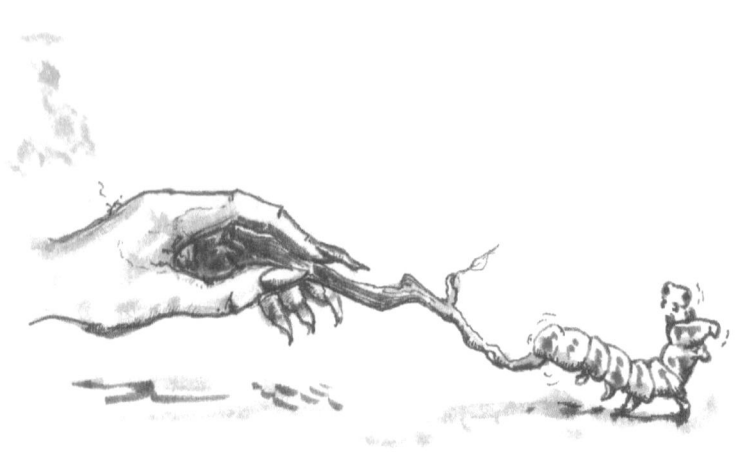

Chapter Twenty: Pushing a Bug with a Stick

I'm holding my stomach while driving down miles and miles of long, dry, desolate road on my way to California to my next travel assignment. My Peter, Paul, and Mary CD's from the 60's are playing over and over again, followed by Alan Jackson's country western songs.

Even though I like the religious hospital I'm

The Yellow "Sick" Road

heading for, the anticipation of this new assignment makes me crazy. At 67 years old, I ask myself, *What the heck am I doing?* I expect that the hospital is going to be herding patients in and out like a cattle drive, because with a capacity of 200, word has it that the turnover is 400 in a month. The reviews are poor, but I need the money for the retirement I have to save for myself because of the jobs I'd lost due to bullying in the workforce.

I'm already homesick and can smell the odor of the motel rooms that are supposedly "No Smoking," the stale towels and sheets, and lumpy mattresses. I've already had the computer training for this job, and now I just need to mentally prepare for taking care of patients. This is what it is all about.

One of the CD'S I was listening to had Alan Jackson singing lyrics to "The Firefly's Song," that went like this:

"I used to go where the devil wouldn't go, where the river run still and the water don't flow, Heaven couldn't stop me then...Good lord willin' and the creek don't rise, and life goes by like the fireflies, where the devil sits with a grin."

Pushing a Bug with a Stick

I've heard it said of me that I used to live on the edge—but I never partook. I ran the Leatherneck Marathon and was in a prominent dance group at BYU (Brigham Young University) called the International Folk Dancers. I thought I could do anything—but my brain and body aren't working quite as quickly these days. I'm still a good nurse because of my twenty-two years of experience and knowledge gained along the way.

In spite of all the days of anticipation for my first day of work, they called me off. This means that they said they didn't need me at that time, so I had to wait for my next scheduled shift to see if I would work. This can happen if their patient load is reduced for some reason.

I hadn't read the small print on the contract, but it said they could call me off once a week for six weeks. Hardly ever on any of my contracts had they called me off. Travel nurses are usually called in because they are desperate and we are needed.

In spite of the kind hospital staff who were happy to answer questions, I was unhappy that they had called me off. I would miss their morning intercom prayer that helped me feel I had a special "something" watching over the patients' and my life. I would miss the environment with the religious statues that offered a feeling of peace.

As the thirteen-week contract played out, I was heartsick that I was repeatedly called off, which only allowed me to work two twelve-hour shifts per week. Out of eleven nurses orientated, they let nine go, leaving only two of us. I'm a good, safe nurse, and they knew it, so they kept me. I was glad I made the cut, but I was bored to tears sitting in the motel room. If I broke the contract and left before it was up, I could be fined $2,500.00. So I waited in the 105 degree California desert heat, grateful that I at least had an air-conditioned motel room.

I felt like an old caterpillar bug pushed by a stick. When pushed, a caterpillar rears up on his hind legs in protest, but when he falls down, the ones holding the stick just keep pushing. Sometimes being an old nurse feels as if I'm the bug and the charge nurse and managers are pushing me with a stick.

While waiting in motel, I read a poem about

Pushing a Bug with a Stick

living in the sixties that described playing with paper dolls, Kick the Can, No Bears Are Out Tonight, riding a stick horse around the house for hours, drawing dot to dot pictures in a coloring book, and looking for empty soda bottles to cash in at the penny candy store to get a tootsie roll. I missed climbing oak trees in the back yard to the tree huts we had built. Life was so simple in those days, little did I know I was ever going to be a nurse. I was so innocent, and so naive.

But I am happy that I now have a real horse named "Flicka," instead of riding my stick horse around the house, and I finally got a check for $9.00 at the barrel race.

How did my life get so hard and complicated?

When the thirteen-week contract was half over, a motel clerk told me I wouldn't be charged any extra to have my dogs stay with me. But after I drove 378 miles home to get my two mini poodles to stay with me so I wouldn't be alone, another clerk told me that I would be charged extra

The Yellow "Sick" Road

for my dogs. Ouch. I drove them home again.

My husband, Scott, stopped by a few times on his truck run to California, which was nice. I also occasionally visited my two sons who lived about an hour and a half's drive from my motel. Sometimes they seemed so busy with their own lives that I felt like an imposition on them.

Another painful poke while in California, I received was a call informing me that my 88-year-old mother had a sudden change in her medical condition. She was unresponsive. I drove all night to visit her at a hospital. I thought she wasn't going to make it, but she rebounded, and after a month and half of hospital care and rehab, she was home and doing well.

The hospital clerk poked me with a very sharp stick by yelling at me for putting the wrong patient's paper in the wrong chart. I know I made a mistake, but she yelled at me in front of everybody, "You just made a Hippa Violation."

Ok, I'm sorry I made a mistake. Please don't yell at me so everybody, including the patients, can hear. I'll fix the problem, and I won't do it again. Write me up or whatever—just please don't humiliate me and yell at me at the nurses station.

In spite of the painful pokes, I survived this contract and made enough money to get me a little more security for my old age.

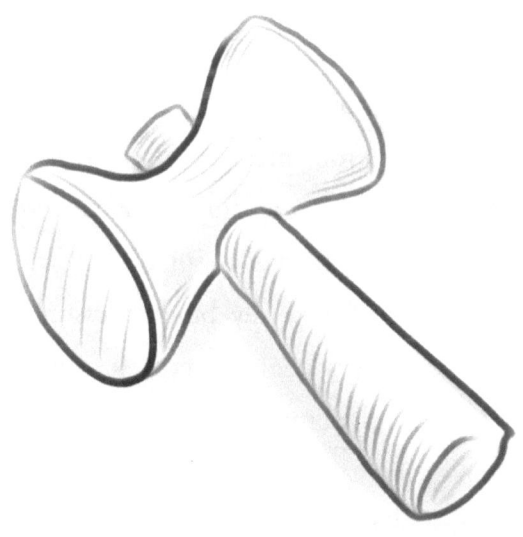

Chapter Twenty-One: Legislature and Statute of Limitations

It may take a village to raise a child, but even more, it takes a legislature to bring reform

I've made it. At this writing, I'm 67 years old and thinking that it may be time to put nursing on the back burner and retire. Do I have enough money saved? If not, will I ever?

Legislature and Statute of Limitations

My last travel assignment to Las Vegas was so stressful that after my shift was over, I took my blood pressure. It was too high to even register. Just knowing I couldn't get a reading made me crazy.

I went to a different hospital's ER clerk and asked if they could take my blood pressure for me. The clerk said they couldn't take it unless I was admitted. I just rolled my eyes and walked away.

I went to my car in the parking lot and lay down, telling myself that at least I was not symptomatic. I had no shortness of breath or chest pain or anything, but I wanted to be close to a hospital just in case. Sleep hit me fast, and I awoke in the morning, glad to know I hadn't died overnight.

I couldn't help thinking that I wouldn't be in this situation if the Big hospital had not laid me off in the unfair manner they did. I'd been in enough other hospitals that I knew things could be run more fairly and with better people skills.

But the facts are the facts. Since mismanagement in the medical field affects not only doctors and nurses, but the general population that uses hospitals, the legislature needs to be aware of the harm done and the abuse that goes unchecked in the medical industry. It seems that because unemployment is so high, some managers take advantage of the large pool of applicants and throw them away for the smallest infraction. Protection needs to be put in place against the Witches who don't know how to treat human beings with fairness or compassion.

CARDINAL RULES AND POLICIES THAT SHOULD BE IMPLEMENTED AT HOSPITALS:

1. Most management has not had any leadership training or experience. Their role is so important that the legislature needs to make it mandatory for management to be trained and certified. What they do and how they interact with employees, patients, and families is crucial. HR (Human Resources) should have equal education and professionalism as the person they are terminating.

2. Management job candidates should have a personality or job description test to see if their personality is management-appropriate.

3. There needs to be a rule against yelling, using abusive gestures in private or public, gossiping, promoting favorite employees without cause, or distributing unfair workloads. Examples:

Legislature and Statute of Limitations

    a. No favoritism given to other nurses so they can make more money by giving them more shifts to work and taking work time away from staff nurses.

    b. Patient assignment should be fair and safe according to patient true acuity. Charge nurses should not give their friends the easy assignments, and no admits and discharges to their favorites.

    c. Every nurse who breaks a rule or policy should be treated equally, and not be bypassed to suffer consequences because of a friendship.

    d. When a lay off is necessary, it should be done by hire date and not by whoever is targeted to be run out.

4. Violation of the above mentioned should result in the offender being ticketed, charged with a misdemeanor, and penalized by a monetary fine.

5. Management should dress and act professionally.

6. All management, CEOS, and employees should sign a contract of policies and consequences related to management and employee fairness laws.

7. Information should be given to employees about abuse so they know whom to contact if it happens. Mandatory workshops should be presented to empower employees with knowledge of the rules and consequences for every employee, from management to first year nurses.

8. There needs to be criteria established for write-ups, where the employee would be warned before termination, and put on probationary status to allow a chance to improve the problem.

9. Discipline should be conducted privately.

10. These cardinal rules shouldn't only apply to employees; they should also apply to customers, vendors, family members, patients, and anyone who hinders a nurse in doing his or her job. Even the top CEO performers should be ticketed and charged with a misdemeanor if their behavior warrants it.

STATUTE OF LIMITATIONS

After finishing my last contract, I was on the phone talking to attorneys for several days to see if I could take any action regarding the episode where the words, "Don't hire Claudia Sanborn" projected over my interviewer's vocera.

Basically, they all said that I had a case. Some of the attorneys were shocked at what happened, but it was past the Statute of Limitations. There was nothing they could do about it now. I tried explaining that if I had acted earlier, I could have been blackballed and never gotten hired anywhere, ever.

Legislature and Statute of Limitations

Be it known that

H.B. 216

Workplace Abusive Conduct Amendments

to Promote a Healthy Workplace

Sponsored by Representative Keven J. Stratton

Co-Sponsored by Senator Todd Weiler

Passed the Utah State Legislature and was signed

by the Speaker of the House and the President of the Senate

In acknowledgment whereof,

I, Gary R. Herbert, Governor of the State of Utah,

affix my signature

to this ceremonial copy of the bill

on May 18, 2015

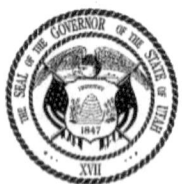

Gary R. Herbert
Governor

They were sympathetic, but the law is the law.

In the Creating a Better Work Environment committee I learned about a nurse who sued a big local hospital. Her picture and name were on the front page of the newspaper. After about a year, she won the case, but nobody would hire her. She was ruined and she knew it. I remember her advising us to not sue because it was a mentally horrible existence and not worth it.

CARDINAL RULE FOR STATUTE OF LIMITATIONS

The judge should determine the time frame for each situation, and be able to interpret the circumstances and state what the time frame should be.

In closing, I'd like to say that one of the best ways to avoid a bullying boss is to not engage them. It is hard to resist reacting and to stay calm and kind and respectful, but that is what can deflect bullying behavior.

Research your job before you take it, because it's

next to impossible to change a lion into a little kitten. What I have learned the hard way is if the company has a reputation of poor management, it is better to not join them in the beginning.

It is hard being a travel nurse because the recruiters are really good at hiding the bad sides of the organizations. Remember that you can't count on trying to change your company or your boss. This doesn't mean that we want a spineless pushover when we need leadership. Disagreement is healthy and needs to happen respectfully in a workplace.

I have used characters from the Wizard of Oz to help you visualize some of the bullying situations I have encountered in my career. The Tin Man, Scarecrow, and Lion represent some of the attributes I've tried to instill to make me a better person as I've traveled the sometimes crooked, sometimes bumpy, and sometimes pleasant Yellow Sick Road.

With all my sincere good intentions,

—Claudia Sanborn RN

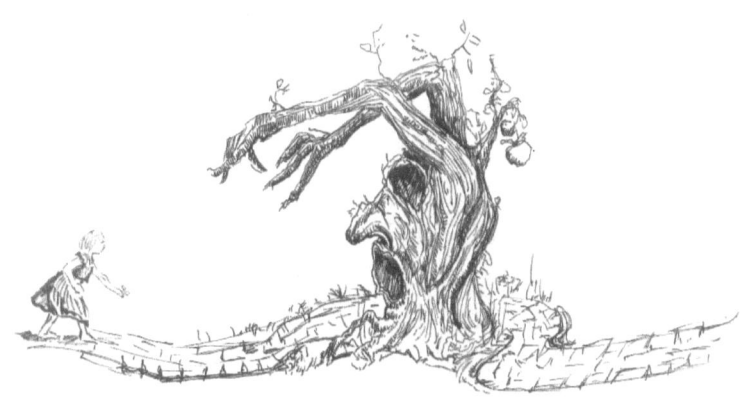

There's an Old Sick Road

On the Yellow Sick Road
Where the sun shines through
By the dark storm clouds
In the mountains of dew

On the Yellow Sick Road
Made strangely sweet
By the touch divine
Of the people we meet

On the Yellow Sick Road
Where my patients are dear
And I walk with them
When the angels are near

On the Yellow Sick Road
With shadows between
I feel myself walk
With the people I meet.

I changed the wording of this ballad, "There's an Old, Old Road," to reflect what I feel as I've traveled along the road of nursing and interacting with patients. It has a beautiful melody that I enjoy playing on my guitar.

Thank you,

—Claudia Sanborn

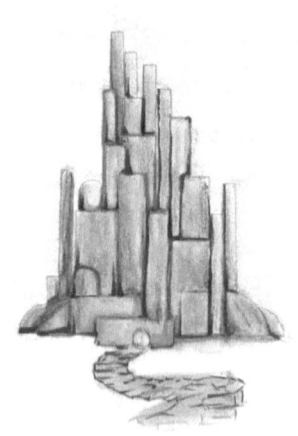

About the Author

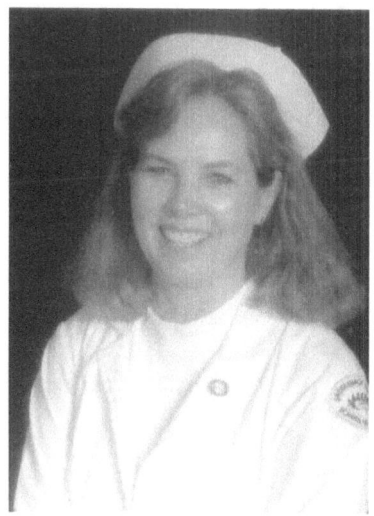

Claudia Sanborn was born and raised in Salt Lake City, Utah. While attending Brigham Young University in 1965, she took some nursing pre-requisite classes.

After marrying, her husband was transferred to Orange County, California in 1980, where Claudia signed up for more nursing classes. She also worked on a Health Science Degree at Chapman University in the City of Orange.

Later, when she became a single parent raising four sons, she was motivated to finish her nursing degree to help support them. It was a difficult hill to climb, but in 1992, she finished her Associated Nursing Degree at Saddleback College.

Traveling the road that wound through the working world of nursing, Claudia soon discovered that it was rather bumpy, crooked, yet sometimes pleasant. When she recognized bullying in the medical field, she started keeping a journal of all the dysfunction she saw in management and administration.

In spite of some traumatic bullying experiences, Claudia continues to work as a nurse. She also participates on the Creating a Better Work Environment committee in Salt Lake City, Utah, that is working toward legislation to make bullying in the workforce illegal.

Besides nursing, Claudia's loves are barrel racing her horse and restoring her 1883 National Historic Registered cabin and pioneer home. This is where she feels, as in the Wizard of Oz, that there's no place like home.

For more information regarding bullying in the workplace, email Claudia Sanborn at: claudiasanborn7@gmail.com.

Acknowledgments

It would take a book in itself to explain what it has been like to write this "Yellow Sick Road" book. It has caused me to reflect, ponder, and soul-search to share these experiences that I have gone through in the last twenty-two years as a nurse. I kept notes in a journal and planned to write this book when I felt I was close to retirement age so I wouldn't get blackballed.

I want to thank my husband, Scott, who would listen to me read a chapter if I made him pancakes for breakfast. The Sanpete Writer's Guild encouraged me and helped the best they could for such an inexperienced writer—but they knew I had a story to tell. Thanks for their comments, especially Steve Clark and for Shirley Bahlmann for editing detail and helping it make sense. Thanks to Kim Jo Smith for her encouragement. Bruce Sanborn, my brother in law, did all the artwork, which really helped me express in pictures what I was trying to say. Thanks to my four sons, Jeff, Ryan, Scott, and Mark, who were there with me through nursing school and my hundreds of flashcards and taped lectures. They have been there through my life, and at times we just held on together, trying to figure it all out.

And thanks to the "Wizard of Oz" book by Frank L. Baum. When I was in Washington, DC, on a nurse travel assignment, I went through the Smithsonian Museum and saw Dorothy's Ruby Slippers. I was so excited to see the actual slippers that I started reading all the books I could find on how "The Wizard of Oz" was written, who wrote it, when it was written, and how all the characters came to be. I related to the "No place like home" sentiment because I missed my "Home, Sweet Home" pioneer house in Utah while on traveling nurse assignments.

My intent is not to be mean or vindictive, but to be blunt to show the need for change starting with Legislation and Policies and Procedures in the medical field.

Here is a quote, which has given me some peace and forgiveness:

"If we could read the secret history of our enemies we would find in each man's sorrow and suffering enough to disarm all hostility."

—Henry Wadsworth Longfellow

Bibliography

[i] Robbins, Alexandra. *The Nurses: A Year of Secrets, Drama, and Miracles with the Heroes of the Hospital.* New York City: Workman, 2015. Print

www.ingramcontent.com/pod-product-compliance
Lightning Source LLC
Chambersburg PA
CBHW030744180526
45163CB00003B/909